Occupational Science

Occupational Science: Society, Inclusion, Participation

Edited by

Gail E. Whiteford
Macquarie University
Sydney, NSW
Australia

Clare Hocking
Auckland University of Technology
Auckland
New Zealand

WILEY-BLACKWELL
A John Wiley & Sons, Ltd., Publication

Blackwell Publishing was acquired by John Wiley & Sons in February 2007. Blackwell's publishing program has been merged with Wiley's global Scientific, Technical and Medical business to form Wiley-Blackwell.

Registered office: John Wiley & Sons, Ltd, The Atrium, Southern Gate, Chichester, West Sussex, PO19 8SQ, UK

Editorial offices: 9600 Garsington Road, Oxford, OX4 2DQ, UK
The Atrium, Southern Gate, Chichester, West Sussex, PO19 8SQ, UK
111 River Street, Hoboken, NJ 07030-5774, USA

For details of our global editorial offices, for customer services and for information about how to apply for permission to reuse the copyright material in this book please see our website at www.wiley.com/wiley-blackwell.

Library of Congress Cataloging-in-Publication Data

Society, inclusion, participation : critical perspectives on occupational science / edited by Gail Whiteford, Clare Hocking.
p. ; cm.
Includes bibliographical references and index.
ISBN-13: 978-1-4443-3316-9 (pbk. : alk. paper)
ISBN-10: 1-4443-3316-X (pbk. : alk. paper)
I. Whiteford, Gail. II. Hocking, Clare.
[DNLM: 1. Occupational Therapy. 2. Social Justice. WB 555]
LC-classification not assigned
615.8′515–dc23 2011030351

A catalogue record for this book is available from the British Library.

Wiley also publishes its books in a variety of electronic formats. Some content that appears in print may not be available in electronic books.

1 2012

Contents

Part III: Ways of knowing occupation

Part IV: Ways of doing in occupational science

Part V: Visioning a way forward

Dedication

We would like to dedicate this book to two leaders who have influenced, guided and mentored us over the years: Professor Ann Wilcock and Professor Elizabeth Townsend. Their scholarship set in train a new consciousness, of global issues such as occupational deprivation and occupational justice, amongst others. By introducing these concepts to the international occupational science community, Ann and Liz have been fundamental to its forward development. Both were prepared to show true leadership – even when it was personally and professionally challenging – and for this we are grateful. Our vision, hopefully realized at least in part through this book, is that there are emerging leaders who will progress their work and entrench its relevance in new places and in multiple contexts.

Gail E. Whiteford and Clare Hocking

About the Editors

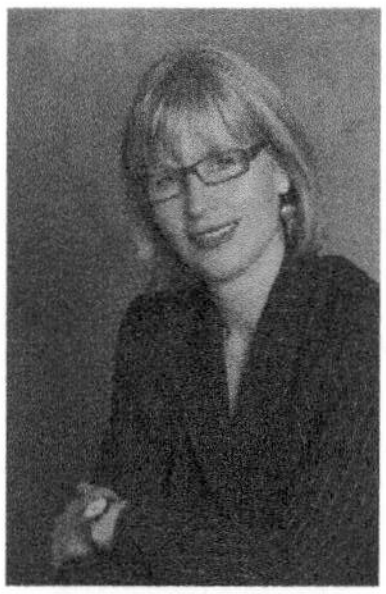

Gail E. Whiteford, PhD
Pro Vice Chancellor (Social Inclusion) Macquarie University, Sydney, NSW, Australia.

Professor Gail Whiteford currently holds the position of Pro Vice Chancellor (Social Inclusion) at Macquarie University, the first position of its type established in Australia. In this position she was invited by the Australian Social Inclusion Unit to speak at the inaugural social inclusion conference in Australia. Gail was a doctoral student of Ann Wilcock and highly influenced by her work, which she extended into her exploration of occupational deprivation and other forms of social exclusion. Gail has been on the Editorial Board of the *Journal of Occupational Science* since 1993 and has numerous publications on occupational science.

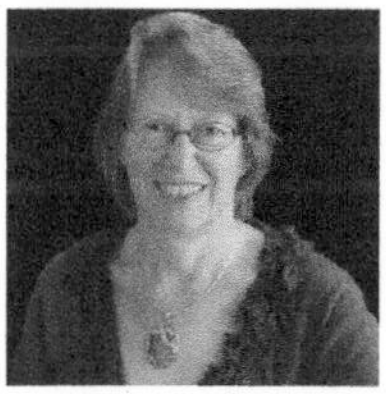

Clare Hocking, PhD
Associate Professor, Department of Occupational Science and Therapy, Faculty of Health and Environmental Sciences, Auckland University of Technology, Auckland, New Zealand.

Best known for her longstanding editorship of the *Journal of Occupational Science*, Clare encountered occupational science as a postgraduate student in Dr Ann Wilcock's papers at the University of South Australia. Inspired by Wilcock's vision, she went on to develop postgraduate papers on occupational science at AUT University in the 1990s. Clare's research has focused on the relationship between the objects people have and use, and their identity, and the cross-cultural meanings of food-related occupations for older women in Thailand, New Zealand and Kentucky, USA. Clare has been an invited keynote speaker and visiting scholar in Australia, Japan, North America and the United Kingdom, and has served as a critical voice in occupational therapy and occupational science over the last 20 years. In this text, Clare's gaze falls on the limited scope of occupational science research.

Contributors

Malcolm P. Cutchin, PhD
Professor of Occupational Science, University of North Carolina at Chapel Hill, NC, USA and University of Southern Denmark, Odense, Denmark

Malcolm's PhD doctorate is in geography. He conducts research at the intersection of social gerontology, occupational therapy and health geography. For almost 20 years, his scholarship has explored the potential of pragmatism for inquiry in those fields.

Silke Dennhardt, MSc
Doctoral candidate, Doctoral Program in Occupational Science, Health and Rehabilitation Sciences, Faculty of Health Sciences, Elborn College, The University of Western Ontario, London, ON, Canada

Silke's experiences of transitioning to a foreign culture raised her awareness of macro-level contexts of occupation and led her to question many of her beliefs. Taking a critical stance, her research focuses on how 'risk' as a particular thinking style, shapes people's occupations and their possibilities to engage in occupation.

Virginia A. Dickie, PhD, OT/L, FAOTA
Associate Professor and Director, Division of Occupational Science and Occupational Therapy, The University of North Carolina at Chapel Hill, Chapel Hill, NC, USA

Virginia's scholarly focus is to build knowledge of occupation in its full complexity. Her ethnographic enquiries into craft production and marketing, and contemporary quilt-making have forced her to see occupation as transactional; involving individuals and groups, technology, materials, place, time, history, culture, politics and more.

Roshan Galvaan, PhD
Senior Lecturer, Division of Occupational Therapy, University of Cape Town, Cape Town, South Africa

Roshan's doctoral thesis investigated a construct fundamental to occupational justice, that is, occupational choice, finding that the nature of occupational choice is contextually situated and population-based. Her continued research explores occupation-based discourses that support the vision of achieving occupational justice for all.

Sarah Kantartzis, MSc
PhD student at Leeds Metropolitan University, Leeds, West Yorkshire, UK. Research Associate at the Centre for Research into Disability and Society, Curtin University, Perth, Western Australia, Australia

Sarah has lived in Greece for 30 years, working as an occupational therapist both in practice and higher education. She is currently undertaking research to explore the nature of occupation and the daily life of adults in a small Greek town.

Elizabeth Anne Kinsella, PhD
Associate Professor, School of Occupational Therapy, Faculty of Health Sciences, Faculty of Education & Women's Studies and Feminist Research, University of Western Ontario, London, ON, Canada; and Adjunct Associate Professor, Research Institute for Professional Practice Learning and Education, Faculty of Education, Charles Sturt University, NSW, Australia

Anne researches processes of reflection, critical reflection and reflexivity in everyday and professional life. Her scholarly interests include the philosophical foundations of social research, epistemologies of practice, professional knowledge, ethics, human occupation, creative arts, end-of-life occupation and occupational identity.

Debbie Laliberte Rudman, PhD
Associate Professor and Faculty Scholar, School of Occupational Therapy and Field Chair, Occupational Science, Graduate Program in Health and Rehabilitation Sciences, The University of Western Ontario, London, ON, Canada

Debbie was introduced to critical social theory as a doctoral student in Public Health Sciences at the University of Toronto. Her work attends to the power relations through which possibilities for occupation are shaped and negotiated, with particular foci on issues related to exclusion, inequity and injustice.

Lilian Magalhães, PhD
Assistant Professor of the School of Occupational Therapy, University of Western Ontario, London, ON, Canada

Lilian is an occupational therapist who was born in Rio de Janeiro, Brazil. She holds a PhD in Public Health from the University of Campinas, Sao Paulo. While in Brazil, in the 1980s, Dr Magalhães studied and worked with participatory and art-based approaches under the supervision of Paulo Freire and Augusto Boal.

Matthew Molineux, PhD
Director of Allied Health, Clinical Education and Training Queensland, Queensland Health, Brisbane Australia and Adjunct Research Fellow, School of Occupational Therapy and Social Work, Curtin University, Perth, Australia

Matthew is an occupational therapist and occupational scientist who has worked as a clinician and academic in Australia and the UK.

Robert B. Pereira, BOccThy (Hons)
PhD Candidate, Centre for Research on Social Inclusion, and Senior Occupational Therapist, Disability Service, Campus Wellbeing Division, Macquarie University, Sydney, NSW, Australia

Robert is interested in the relationship between social inclusion policy and the experience of living with multiple disadvantages. His clinical and research interests include social inclusion, health promotion, chronic disease management, policy analysis, narrative inquiry and occupational justice.

Ben Sellar, BOccThy (Hons)
PhD Candidate, Centre for Research into Social Inclusion, Macquarie University, Sydney, and Lecturer, Occupational Therapy Program, University of South Australia, Adelaide, Australia

Ben worked as an occupational therapist in therapeutic and community development roles with children who have experienced domestic violence, and now teaches community development and occupational science. His current research focuses on justice, subjectivity, politics, science and critical methodologies.

Alison Wicks, PhD
University of Wollongong, Nowra, NSW, Australia

Alison is the Founding Director of the Australasian Occupational Science Centre and Senior Lecturer in Occupational Science at the Shoalhaven Campus of the University of Wollongong. She is a Board member of the International Society for Occupational Science and President of the Australasian Society of Occupational Scientists.

Valerie A. Wright-St Clair, PhD
Senior Lecturer, School of Rehabilitation and Occupation Studies, and Co-Director of the Active Ageing Research Cluster, Person Centred Research Centre, Auckland University of Technology, Auckland, New Zealand

Valerie's research spans gerontology, occupational science, cross-cultural research and interpretive phenomenology. Her focus is in how elders' participation in everyday activities influences longevity, health and wellness; elders' integration and participation within communities, and understanding the meaning of what people do.

Preface

Schooled by Ann Wilcock to appreciate the power of occupation to promote health and well-being, we have been passionate supporters of the development of occupational science for almost two decades. This book is an expression of that passion. It is offered as a critical reflection, in appreciation of what occupational science might become and the influence it might have on the future of human and ecological health.

The spirit of the book is critical. It brings together established and emerging voices in the discipline to offer diverse perspectives on the development of occupational science and the realities to which occupational scientists are attuned. Some of the critique we offer has been previously voiced – for example, the concentration of effort on understanding individual rather than collective experience and the western orientation of the research effort. In this volume, such concerns are given new depth and breadth through the author's extended consideration. Other perspectives are newly voiced: the ideological positions taken up by occupational scientists, the way risk discourses shape engagement in occupation, and ways socio-economic and political realities shape the occupational choices of South African youths.

Critique is unfamiliar territory for many of us. Rather, our concern with the nature and potential of occupation is expressed in a spirit of exploration, an uncovering of new insights, the excitement of fresh understandings. We turn to our participants for confirmation of findings, and to each other for acknowledgement that our ideas are ground-breaking, rich, and insightful. That positive critique is invaluable. It energises researchers to continue in their work, and encourages new comers to seek opportunities to make their own contribution.

Criticism without challenge, however, supports complacency and limits potential for growth. It fails both scholars and researchers in neglecting opportunities to hone their ideas, uncover the assumptions limiting their insights, and recognise the boundaries to their vision. It creates a culture where no-one asks the hard questions: What is important to know? How can that knowledge be applied to secure an occupationally just future? In offering this critique, we trust that readers will join us in valuing the opinions expressed and the arguments advanced. Constructive criticism can generate respect within a community committed to reaching forward to a better future. A community that encompasses honest attempts to express criticism and doubt, despite the discomfort, opens the door to seeing the bigger picture, and making a difference.

Our hope is that you will be challenged, informed and inspired by this book. We willingly acknowledge that many other perspectives might have been brought to bear, and that we have not represented all of the critical voices in the field. Rather, this is a work in progress, a point in time. We look forward to being part of the new conversations that the ideas expressed in this volume unleash. To close, we acknowledge those who willingly accepted our invitation to contribute to this collection by sharing a traditional Maori proverb:

> Ui mai koe ki ahau he aha te mea nui o te ao, Māku e kī atu he tangata, he tangata, he tangata!
> Ask me what is the greatest thing in the world, I will reply: It is people, it is people, it is people!

Gail E. Whiteford
Clare Hocking
2011

Part I

Introduction

Introduction to critical perspectives in occupational science

1

Clare Hocking and Gail E. Whiteford

Introduction

Occupational Science: Society, Inclusion, Participation advances an emancipatory agenda in which we stress the power of occupation to address global population inequities. The agenda is informed by a suite of initiatives undertaken by local governments, non-government organizations and individual citizens working to improve the lives of vulnerable people. Such initiatives include, amongst others, those aimed at income creation for persons excluded from labour markets, developing safe environments following natural disasters, and reducing the impact of infectious diseases including AIDS, tuberculosis and malaria through community-based education programmes.

As occupational scientists, we have framed the ideas presented in this book relative to such global initiatives in explicitly occupational terms. Examples of populations with occupational needs include people excluded from education and work that would ensure their survival and provide the means to rise out of poverty, people participating in antisocial and self-destructive occupations, and those forced into degrading and

Occupational Science: Society, Inclusion, Participation, First Edition.
Edited by Gail Whiteford and Clare Hocking.

life-threatening occupations (e.g., slave labour, forced prostitution). Examples of phenomena cast in occupational terms include:

- Environmental degradation caused through patterns of occupational participation that are inappropriate to their specific context;
- The disruption of traditional occupations in discrete communities and the corollaries of this;
- The increasing burden of caregiving in communities at one end of the spectrum affected by population diseases such as HIV/AIDS, and at the other end because of increased life expectancy;
- The continued occupational deprivation experienced by populations affected by natural disasters and conflicts;
- The mobilization of oppressed and marginalized groups into civic action as a response to the exclusions and occupational injustices they have experienced.

Our hope, in assembling the collection of critical essays presented here, has been to stimulate the development of a more critical and reflexive science of occupation. Through the examination and illumination of the ontological biases and assumptions that currently limit our science, we challenge the reader to re-think what may be taken for granted in their own work. Such a reflexive stance enables the possibility of a more socially responsive discipline which in turn is able to make robust and relevant contributions to societal reform, inclusion and participation. To achieve this admittedly ambitious aim, we assembled a range of critical perspectives that would inspire, guide and inform knowledge development salient to an active engagement with pressing societal issues of an essentially occupational nature.

Chapter authors were invited to address the underlying societal structures and the occupational injustices that prevent inclusion and participation, from the perspective of their own practice, research and scholarship. Our hope is that their ideas set new parameters and directions for the development of occupational science into the future. With this objective in mind, the book begins with Magalhães' exposition on oppression and liberation in which she invokes the wisdom of her Brazilian mentor, Paulo Freire. Her reflection problematizes the very nature of occupational science, highlighting attendant tensions between an essential humanism and an at times positivist epistemology. Pointing to issues of language, science and power, Magalhães' interrogates the risk of accepting the reductionist and individualistic perspective of biomedical science, rather than the emancipatory and collectivist agenda that Freire advanced. Set in a real-world context that acknowledges the personal costs of activism, her lively contribution reminds us of the necessity of theorizing social action in order to understand the purposes it ultimately serves.

Understanding occupation, the second section of the book, presents an ontological grounding for the ways occupational scientists might best conceptualize people's engagement in occupation. Citing the predominance of an individualist perspective in occupational science research, even in studies that investigated group-based occupations, Cutchin and Dickie examine the limitations of a science that conceptualizes humans as individual agents responsive to their own needs and meanings. Informed by Dewey's understanding of human experience as embedded in particular situations, they firmly place human endeavours within a transactional framework that supports improvement in people's lives by reconstructing established customs and institutions. In advocating Dewey's pragmatist attitude, Cutchin and Dickie focus on three dimensions of action: habits – which restrict the participation of people living in restricted circumstances, context – which contains multiple possibilities for action, and creativity – which is required to inquire into and reconfigure habits that will enable the growth of individuals and communities for the common good. As Cutchin and Dickie emphasize, the process of engaging with the world is always a shared inquiry.

Furthering that work, Kantartzis and Molineux critique the genesis and development of occupational science. It is, they assert, predominantly anglophonic in its orientation, and thus informed by the religious, economic, political and educational ideas that have shaped the Western world. Invoking Foucault's warning that the context from which knowledge emerges has important consequences for the possibilities it might envisage, they remind us that uncritiqued understandings generally represent and reinforce individualized experiences of reality. Consequently, the assumptions about the patterns, norms and meanings of daily occupations that are familiar to people in the English-speaking world do not align with other world views and cultural constructions. Such a disjunction, they suggest, limits the relevance and expansion of occupational science in the future. Illustrating their argument, Kantartzis and Molineux draw from an ethnographic study of daily life in a small Greek village. Their work reveals a flexible interweaving of familial, social and productive occupations inconceivable in post-industrialized settings in which work as a basis of identity construction and social location is more common.

Reflecting further on the limitations of Eurocentric perceptions of the nature of occupation, Hocking picks up and extends previous critiques of occupational science as being essentially individualistic in orientation, emphasizing individual experiences of everyday occupations rather than the ways they shape and are shaped by groups and communities. Occupational scientists' narrow focus on socially sanctioned occupations and a feminized lens on occupations of significance are also critiqued as ontological perspectives that constrain the field's contribution to critical scholarship and processes of social change.

Kinsella's account of occupational scientists as an epistemic community opens the third section of the book, *Ways of knowing occupation*. Drawing on Kuhn's assertion that scientists make judgements about the utility of theories based on shared epistemic values, Kinsella describes how theory choice, and thus knowledge development, in occupational science is determined by perceptions of the accuracy, simplicity, scope, fruitfulness and consistency of the theories it adopts and rejects. Since individuals might make different judgements, even in relation to the same criteria, it is the shared judgement of the community that effectively decides the field's theoretical direction. These considerations are important, because such values influence the possibilities for and approaches taken to knowledge generation. On that basis, Kinsella urges the adoption of technical, practical and emancipatory knowledge paradigms and diverse criteria for knowledge claims in occupational science.

The implicit judgement behind this book is the necessity of a critical perspective on occupational science, which is the focus of Sellar's discussion. Characterizing the field's current critical stance as Marxian, he argues that theorists have pitted the natural occupational predispositions of humans against unjust societal practices and policies that alienate people from their needs. That is, occupational science has separated 'natural laws' (the biological needs and drives that underpin health) from human beliefs and values (which obscure what people need and give rise to injustices). Sellar argues that rather than merely extending that critique, occupational scientists should embrace understandings more suited to occupational science's perspective on human existence. In so doing, they would be freed to consider what it really means to be critical and what critical practices make possible.

One critical perspective proposed by Laliberte Rudman explores how expectations and possibilities for occupation are shaped by social and political processes. To inform her argument, Laliberte Rudman draws on both critically informed life course perspectives and governmentality theory, which draw attention to complex contextual influences on the ways in which entrée into patterns of occupational participation are made easier for dominant groups whilst excluding or marginalizing others. In addressing the ways occupation is governed, her critical analysis points to cultural, political and structural causations. While acknowledgement of the importance of context is not new, most occupational science research continues to overlook the social processes and mechanisms through which occupational injustices are created and become entrenched as taken for granted practices. Laliberte Rudman maps out a critical approach intended to open up possibilities for dialogue and action towards human flourishing.

Of course, there are also discourses which delimit human flourishing. Dennhardt, in a chapter written in partnership with Laliberte Rudman, introduces risk as such a discourse and explores it from an occupational perspective, a relatively new contribution to the occupational science literature. How occupational scientists frame risk and relate it to occupation will inform possible actions and solutions in relation to occupations deemed as high risk and with respect to at-risk populations. As Dennhardt and Laliberte argue, however, risk is connected to power, in that defining risk preempts the responses viewed as rational and possible. Risk, they argue, is alternately framed as an objective hazard that can be quantified, predicted and controlled by rational agents acting on expert advice, or as unanticipated, uncontrollable and socially constructed, albeit with real impacts on individuals and society. Given the pervasive nature and impacts of the risk discourse, and the hegemonic practice that often accompanies it, an occupational science research agenda in this area seems requisite.

Following on from these discussions of the nature of occupation and the perspectives from which it might be viewed, the fourth section of the book addresses more practical concerns; *Ways of doing in occupational science*. The first consideration in endeavouring to understand the complexity of vulnerable people's occupations and occupational needs, and the occupational justice issues affecting people internationally, is the choice of research methodology. As Wright-St. Clair argues, how we might come to know occupation in its fullness and determining how human occupation ought to be measured are challenging questions. Underpinning those questions are considerations of the meaning of being a science, what counts as occupational science research, and whether the field is best served by unconstrained organic growth or more focused exploration of pressing social questions. Espousing the value of multiple research methodologies to address different kinds of research questions, Wright-St. Clair also points out that science encompasses the development and application of theory and identification of phenomena of interest.

One phenomenon of interest, in relation to equity of access and occupational justice, is the occupational choices people perceive as being open to them. Galvaan's study, which involved young adolescents in a marginalized community in Cape Town, South Africa, employed critical ethnographic methods of inquiry. Against the backdrop of forced relocation into racially segregated communities in the 1970s, that are now characterized by poverty, unemployment, overcrowding, violence, poor access to recreational opportunities and low educational attainment, Galvaan explored participants' occupational choices over four years. In making sense of the ways the youths' occupational patterns perpetuated historical injustices, she identified political and socio-economic influences that both constrained and enabled occupation, describing how choices were constructed in transaction with the environment. That is, the participants' context was more than a backdrop to occupational choice; it was part of the choices they made, contingent on their experience of historically and politically determined patterns of occupation and style of housing, the subcultures they were part of, and others' low educational expectations of them.

From this locally situated example of engaging in occupation the discussion moves to the international stage, with Wicks' critique of the role the International Society of Occupational Science (ISOS) has played in fostering the development of the field. Bringing together the need for a coherent, widely adopted knowledge of human occupation and her vision of the ISOS's potential role, Wicks envisages a respected, sustainable representative body that is well placed to influence policy, participation and practice. Evidencing movement towards that vision, Wicks documents a shift within occupational science, from primarily focusing on occupation's role in health to the broader issues of occupational justice and advocacy. ISOS has been instrumental in bringing that re-visioning about, influencing the formulation and adoption of a Position Statement on Human Rights by the World Federation of Occupational Therapists. Going forward, ISOS is setting the stage for the incorporation of international perspectives in the development of occupational science, through its valuing of inclusiveness, multidisciplinarity and diversity and leadership in bringing the occupational science community into dialogue.

The theme of dialogue is extended in the final chapter by Whiteford and Pereira in which they recommend that occupational science engage in a conceptual dialogue with other disciplines. The purpose of this, they suggest, would be to better understand the utility of core concepts and constructs which have developed in occupational science over time. In particular, they suggest that notions of inclusion and participation are particularly salient to such a process, pointing out the close nexus between framings developed within occupational science and elsewhere. At a time when social inclusion has become a driver in policy development internationally, this is a timely critique. In the chapter they also highlight how the ideals of justice and inclusion can be understood through the presentation and discussion of data from Pereira's study of poverty and multiple disadvantage. Their conclusion is that occupational science, in particular constructions of occupational justice which foreground difference and diversity in capabilities, has a substantive contribution to make across the arenas of disability, health and welfare. This is, however, a contribution which has yet to be realized.

2 What would Paulo Freire think of occupational science?

Lilian Magalhães

Who was Paulo Freire and why might he be important to occupational scientists?

Paulo Reglus Neves Freire was born in Recife, Brazil on 19 September 1921. He died on 2 May 1997. His work provided a seminal discussion of the ways in which education is implicated in the dynamics of oppression and liberation. Freire became widely known for his book *Pedagogy of the Oppressed*, which was first published in Portuguese in 1970 and then in English in 1972. His approach to education is deeply rooted in the radical movements for social change that occurred in the 1960s and 1970s and can be aligned with such works as Ivan Illich's (1973) *Deschooling Society*. According to Peter Roberts (2000), Freire's ideas about adult literacy programmes for impoverished workers in Brazil cost him almost 14 years in exile during the military authoritarian rule.

Along with many other scholars, Feinberg and Torres (2001) articulated the connection between the work of this Brazilian educator and John Dewey's tenets of democracy, as well as the undeniable relationship between politics and education. These authors stress the legacy of Freire's works for educators around the globe, which may be clearly seen through the innumerable contexts in which his work has been

Occupational Science: Society, Inclusion, Participation, First Edition.
Edited by Gail Whiteford and Clare Hocking.

applied not only in popular education, but also in health promotion and community development (Wallerstein & Freudenberg, 1998; Yoo, 2007).

Dialogue, Reflection, Practice (which translates into Praxis) and Consciousness-Raising (Conscientização)[1] are essentially the key concepts of Freire's work. The latter is rather a complex concept originally coined in Portuguese, which is difficult to translate into the English language. Nevertheless, it is usually translated as *consciousness-raising*, although without Freire's agreement. In fact, in my opinion, many of the difficulties with the various translations of Freire's works are due not only to semantic differences in language but also to contextual contrasts that may create dissonances between readers. Freire published 37 books during his lifetime and another seven or eight were released after his passing in 1997, taken from unfinished material that he left with his wife, Nita Freire, and friends. It is important to note that Freire wrote entirely in Portuguese and that his books have been translated into at least 35 languages, according to the Paulo Freire Institute, in Brazil. For example, while reflecting on the impact of Freire's work for society in South Korea, the Philippines and Mexico, Yoo (2007) highlighted that 'his radical thought on educational transformation has challenged other social terrains including grassroots human rights movements, environmental (ecological preservation) movements, social welfare and health movements, peace settlement movements in the world, as well as systematic formal school reforms' (Yoo, 2007, p. 81).

Despite his incontestable influence worldwide, Freire has been criticized on many fronts. Feinberg and Torres (2001) reminded us that the Swiss educator Pierre Furter defined Freire as 'a myth in his own lifetime' (p. 61) and, in spite of being a worldwide icon, Freire has endured many criticisms such as having a rather too simplistic view of the dynamics of power. According to Facundo's interpretation, 'one is either an oppressor or oppressed. His rigid structuralist view of the world does not allow for its complexity' (Facundo, 1984, p. 3).

In addition, it has been argued that Freire's popularity was not achieved without some degree of misrepresentation of his proposals and ideas:

> *Not only is there confusion between the man and the myth, but we no longer know whether the ideas we associate with him are to be counted among his intentions, his practical achievements, his successes or his failures, or whether they are simply what he has come to represent in the minds of his contemporaries... It is as though he were regarded as a guru whose message offers a solution to problems of which he is not even aware. What is happening is that Freire is being turned into a kind of fetish, as witness the interest in his "method," his "conscientization," his "system," as though he were offering a universal panacea.* (Furter, 1985, p. 301)

Yet, Freire's importance for those who strive for justice and social change is undeniable and despite the backlash resulting from several of the projects that have claimed his

[1] Traditionally it has been translated as *consciousness-raising* but, in Portuguese, it holds a sense of an insightful process, a kind of critical social awareness that arises from the courageous reflection of one's oppressive lived reality. As Freire stated: 'It is only when the oppressed find the oppressor out and become involved in the organized struggle for their liberation that they begin to believe in themselves. This discovery cannot be purely intellectual but must involve action; nor can it be limited to mere activism, but must include serious reflection: only then will it be a praxis.' (1972, p. 52)

guidance, it is not difficult to find accounts in which Freire's wisdom makes all the more sense even to this day. A very creative book compiled by Sonia Nieto, a long-time friend of Freire's, brings letters from education students who begin their reading of Freire's work. As per Sonia's suggestion, the letters were a way for the students to talk directly to him. The result is a heartfelt, critical and inspiring collection of exchanges that might be summarized by this piece:

> *Paulo, on the late nights, in the rain, when I'm depressed about urban schooling and yet thrilled by the questions of children and adolescents, when the possibilities of rippling social movements are, at once, seemingly endless and impossible to envision, you've gotten me through.* (Michelle Fine, in Nieto, 2008, p. 82)

Thus, as occupational science's body of scholarly works grows, it makes sense to attempt to hold a candid conversation with Freire concerning the main points of convergence between his struggle against oppression and some of the dilemmas of our field.

Why should I write a letter to Freire?

Paulo Freire loved writing and receiving letters. A significant portion of his work was conducted in epistolary exchanges. Starting at the time when he was first in exile, his primary form of communication was by post. Freire's letters were a way to maintain his connections with his family, his friends and his students around the world and Freire utilized this form of exchange extensively (Freire, 1996). Or as Adriano Vieira stated: Freire pursued a dialogue that builds 'in a systematic way, yet [is] warmly human, a rigorous reflection of education issues' (Vieira, 2008, p. 72, original in Portuguese). As in Freire's letters, my correspondence reflects a personal commentary on prevailing conditions.

Where should I begin?

Dear Paulo,

'My friend, you have no idea of the wave of memories now crashing against me …'

(Nise da Silveira, 1999, p. 39, original in Portuguese).

It is difficult for me to express to you how excited and yet ambivalent I have felt as I prepared myself to write this letter. If I could summarize, it has been sweet but somewhat bitter, bright yet dark, reassuring and yet, at the same time, confusing.

First, in case you are already wondering, let me tell you what this project is and why I accepted it. As I will attempt to explain to you later, fate[2] caused me to emigrate to

[2] We know it was not fate, but can we just pretend that it was?

Canada in 2004, and my life has changed considerably since you and I last spoke. In fact, our lives have been greatly changed since we last heard your warm voice illuminating us with your wisdom. As I progress with this letter, I will try to give you a very brief account of our biggest concerns at this point in time. But, for now, it is enough to say that you are sadly missed and that every so often your name comes up in conversations, in publications and at meetings, with all of us wondering how you could assist us in our struggle to respond meaningfully to the current, almost universal, social upheaval. Now, the somewhat comic element here is that, despite the fact that we are both Brazilians and that I have significant English language limitations, I will attempt to write this letter in English, for the reasons that I will later provide.

More to the point: I now hold the position of an assistant professor at the University of Western Ontario, in London, Ontario, Canada. I know that it does not make any sense, but at a certain point in my life the Brazilian context was driving me crazy. Or rather, it was making me bitter. Hence, I decided to enter into a form of voluntary exile. I know how surprised you probably are because you were *forced* into exile during the military rule of the 1960s and, although you made the best out of your 13 years outside your native country, Brazil, it was quite painful for you to abandon your people, your home and your loved ones and to lose the opportunity to speak our beloved Portuguese language and eat our delicious *feijoadas*.[3]

Nevertheless, for me, in spite of the inescapable hardship, emigration appeared to be the best option. So, with five of our wonderful Brazilian poets' books in my suitcase, I arrived in Canada in June 2004, to experience one of the most creative and challenging periods of my life to date despite the *saudade*.[4]

Although you may not remember, I am very proud to be an occupational therapist. You were always very interested in the stories that we, occupational therapists, had to share with you. Of course, it is possible that your attentiveness was partly due to your infectious kindness and your considerable inquisitiveness. But I also remember that you were very curious about a profession that strives to treat people by means of their daily occupations. And, more than once, I remember that we talked about the concept of *praxis* and what it would entail with respect to the effort to generate personal and social change by reflecting about what people do and how they go about doing ordinary things.

As you can see, I tend to digress. But the main point here is that my coming to Canada introduced me to a new discipline called occupational science. That's right, it is a science that has been around for the last two decades, which has experienced various degrees of institutionalization and progress around the globe, and this has been changing the face of occupational therapy in particular in some countries, and to some degree, certain aspects of other human sciences as well. Occupational science was first created to provide occupational therapy with a much-needed and more rigorous

[3] A traditional Brazilian dish made of black beans and pork meat.

[4] '*Saudade* is a Portuguese and Galician word for a feeling of nostalgic longing for something or someone that one was fond of and which is lost. *Saudade* is generally considered one of the hardest words to translate. It originated from the Latin word *solitatem* (loneliness, solitude), but developed a different meaning. Few other languages in the world have a word with such meaning, making *saudade* a distinct mark of Portuguese culture.' (retrieved from search.com)

profile; to be 'a basic science devoted to the study of the human as an occupational being' (Yerxa, 1993, p. 5).

Occupational science has brought a tremendous amount of scholarly discussion to the health care arena. At one point, one of the most influential scholars in the field, a colleague from Australia, Gail Whiteford, asked me: 'Lilian, what would Paulo Freire think of occupational science?' And here I am, several months later, struggling to find a reasonable response.

Professor, I should probably start by telling you that choosing a name for this new science was not easy and the issue is still under scrutiny. The goal of occupational science is to move forward the scientific status of the study of human occupations. I assure you that at least one important founder of the occupational science movement, a North American by the name of Elizabeth Yerxa (2009), is not comfortable with this title, as she questioned:

> *Should occupational science be called a science or be renamed using a broader term such as occupational inquiry? Certainly, if science means integral science as defined earlier, the term science is appropriate. However, if science is defined as reductionistic, narrow thinking, then it is not appropriate.* (p. 495)

Actually, Yerxa went on to discuss the risks of an occupational science that overlooks the complexities of *human consciousness and experience* in order to expand its influence: 'As an occupational scientist and occupational therapist, I have seen the *it* mentality gain prominence in the science and practice of our field as the profession emulates other sciences and responds to pressures to prove its efficacy' (2009, p. 490).

In fact, you, too, have been warning us about the underpinnings of naming and re-naming of the world (Freire, 1972). You have warned us that

> *...the naming of the world, which is an act of creation and re-creation, is not possible if it is not infused with love... It is thus necessarily the task of responsible subjects and cannot exist in a relation of domination.* (p. 89)

I will try to elaborate on this topic later, but I am under the impression that you would see lots of room for discussion about the need for adjectives to accompany the noun *science*, and I would love to hear what you have to say about it. Do you think that we can rescue science from the reductionist proselytism that has been perversely hegemonic in just renaming the fields rather than democratically creating new ones? Is there a risk that by labelling this new field of study as a science, we lose control over its complex roots and come to embrace a soulless discipline? That would be the *it science* that worried Yerxa (2009). Is science always an oppressive social exchange?

However, I wonder if there is such a thing as controlling knowledge and its trajectory? I am certain that we all see the clear relationship between power and science, but will just changing the terminology (names) grant us the emancipatory knowledge for which the practitioners of occupational science may have been longing? Furthermore, I did note that you have used the word *knowledge* far more often than the word *science* and that you greatly dislike the way in which we toss words about in academic circles:

When I think about the language I use and the language the students use when they first come to the university, I have to think again of the dichotomy between reading words and reading the world, between the dance of concepts, a conceptual ballet we learn in the university, and the concrete world that the concepts should be referring to. (Shor & Freire, 1987, p. 147)

My dear professor, I see many signs of light in your writings regarding these issues. Every time I read your discussions about naming the world I cannot help but notice that you speak about language in at least two senses: firstly the power of changing language in order to change reality. As you wrote:

It is not pure idealism; let it be further observed, to refuse to await a radical change in the world in order to begin to insist on a change in language. Changing language is part of the process of changing the world. (Freire, 1994, p. 56)

But also, you referred to the need to keep language connected to everyday life. To be fair, here I must add that the term occupational science may have resulted from the actions of what Henry Giroux (2004, p. 205) described as *transformative intellectuals.* In fact, the term was born out of the work of seriously engaged scholars. And although it was initially received with some criticism, the choice of such a term was certainly not intended to convey an elitist initiative. You have pointed out how important it is and it might be worthwhile to remember how Antonio Gramsci contrasted the social commitments of *organic* and *traditional* intellectuals and 'the key to the creation of counter-hegemonic action' through socially responsible intellectual enterprise (Mayo, 1999, p. 53). The profound influence that Gramsci's work had on your own convictions is clear and I am certain that you would appreciate if occupational scientists would further this discussion: 'I read Gramsci and I discovered that I had been greatly influenced by Gramsci long before I had read him' (Freire, as cited by Mayo, 1999, p. 7).

Actually, in focusing on the commitment of intellectuals to bring about social change, Fischman and McLaren (2005) wrote an excellent paper, which revisited your legacy. They also compared your works to those of Gramsci. And they did a marvellous job of highlighting some of the misappropriations of your (and Gramsci's) works. The main point being, the relationship between theory and practice and the intellectual's responsibility to align these two concepts. As Fischman and McLaren posited: 'Gramsci, like Paulo Freire years later, urged intellectuals to develop a relational knowledge of and with the masses to help them become self-reflective' (p. 433).

Moreover, they revisited your own words:

...conscientization is not exactly the starting point of commitment. Conscientization is more of a product of commitment. I do not have to be already critically self-conscious in order to struggle. By struggling I become conscious/aware. (Freire, 1989, as cited by Fischman & McLaren, 2005, p. 440)

Thus, not surprisingly, because political engagement is a highly controversial subject, the element of social commitment of occupational scientists has been a matter of much discussion. Some scholars envision an unavoidable global political praxis (Thibeault, 2002; Yerxa, 2009) while others might suggest that the claim of universalism in occupational science, namely the imposition of certain Western values, should be viewed with caution as Hammell (2011) stated:

> *...it is difficult to avoid the impression that theories of occupation "belong" to white, middle-class, English-speaking Western theorists and it is important to recall that the area of the world self-designated Western, first or developed, constitutes only about 17% of the global population.* (p. 31)

The universality of our assumptions is obviously a very important debate but somehow, in my opinion, it is yet to be articulated in broader (truly global) terms within occupational science. As it stands at this point, I have some discomfort with the black and white discussion (almost exclusively driven by Western scholars, I must add) that neglects to unpack layers of contemporary hybridity and power intricacies. To put it another way, I am quite glad to see this discussion finally brought to light, but, in my view, a more nuanced analysis is still to be done in order, for example, to uncover concepts such as the myth of a monolithic *white hegemony* (see the recent body of work trying to unpack whiteness) and the power struggles within the so-called *minority world.* I am quite concerned about the risk of certain tokenism in this discussion, which, again, would patronize and stereotype non-westerners.

My dear professor, there are so many points about which I would love to gain your insights. The global context has been atrocious, to say the least. This is not to say that global circumstances have declined in the last decade but to comment on the fact that they have not improved. That fact alone suggests that we are turning around in circles, even though we have accumulated an abundance of theoretical and empirical tools with which to address the issues of poverty and inequality. In fact, I must warn you that we have been distracted by an *absolute* explosion of information, which was engendered by internet technologies and by a media-saturated style of social life that has become globally endemic. As we adapt ourselves to new forms of communication (but not to meaningful dialogue, I am afraid) our occupations have been profoundly changed. My belief is that you would dislike this trend as strongly as I do. To me, it is very worrisome that the activity, which we sometimes address as *education*, is instead merely the transferring of *information* – that is, alienating, thoughtless and biased *information.* We seem to have lost the ability to distinguish between the two concepts.

Hence, we may be being excessively informed, but not really educated. Tons of fragmented information is readily accessible to some of us. But yet, they do not reflect our everyday realities[5] and we are confronted with idealized models of being and doing, which are out of reach for the majority and are often openly dismissive of responsible social engagement.

My dear Paulo, you may be glad to know that there are many concepts on which occupational scientists have been working in order to advance a socially committed

[5] In fact, our TV channels have been inundated by the so-called *reality shows*. This is a type of public exposition of ordinary people through the media, where the least desirable of human characteristics is actually presented as the reality, and in which individualistic and self-indulgent behaviours are celebrated and even openly encouraged.

agenda such as occupational justice (Townsend & Wilcock 2004), occupational deprivation (Whiteford, 2000; Wilcock, 1998), and occupational apartheid (Kronenberg, Algardo, & Pollard, 2005). You may be pleased to learn that social commitment is inseparable from the trajectory of occupational science described above, despite some of its internal tensions. In fact, it has been reassuring to see that many aspects of social exclusion and oppression, which have arisen through the concept of meaningful occupation, have been uncovered by occupational science researchers (Whiteford, 2000).

As an example, in my work with an international group of dedicated colleagues,[6] we have been focusing on what we have described as occupational hardship. It is the type of social, political and economic conditions endured by undocumented immigrants living in large North American cities such as Toronto, in Canada. Silenced by the need to remain invisible, these immigrants may live underground for years and years, performing regular social activities such as working, parenting and contributing through community volunteerism while keeping their identities hidden. This form of existence transforms every move they make into a sophisticated exercise in dissimulation. Occupational science concepts have been vital in our research in this field.

I cannot stress strongly enough how inspiring it would be to have you participate in our humble projects, with your infectious laugh and your courteous but sharp ways of questioning our postulations. Lastly, in the interest of time, in this letter I will focus on one crucial question that requires your urgent consideration and which is the subject of a current debate concerning our profession. It relates to *individual-based* contrasted to *socially focused* interventions. In recent scholarly work this tension can be summarized as the opposition between *individual agency* and *collective action* (Kronenberg, Pollard, & Sakellariou, 2011; Reid, 2011).

Dear professor, have you altered your previous arguments? As I remember, you made quite clear your conviction concerning the importance of conscientization and the necessity of that process being a collective pursuit. As your long-time friend Sonia Nieto reminded us: 'To him [Paulo Freire], it was, above all, a social process that went beyond the mere seizing of consciousness' (Nieto, 2008, p. 89). As difficult as the translation of your work from Portuguese to English is, as I mentioned before, I have no hesitation in remarking on your collective perspective that is so clearly evidenced throughout your writings. Nieto revisited your conviction to clarify the matter: 'Further, he also declared "I am more and more convinced that the word should really be used in the Brazilian form, conscientização, and spelled that way"' (Freire, n.d. as cited by Nieto, 2008, p. 89).

Professor, a positivistic frame has been at the core of health care for as long as we all can recall. While building a discipline that strives to relate the concept of occupation to the ideals of health and wellness, occupational scientists are sometimes seduced by the appealing objectivity of the individual perspective. Even if one cannot deny the importance of *context* in ordinary human activities, the ever-present dilemma of measurability haunts us as does a mermaid's chant.

Many recent works have corroborated the importance of social engagement. Yet, in my opinion, we very often fail to understand the impossibility of full emancipation in individual terms. In fact, individual aspects of a human life cannot replace social interaction. In your episteme, you often reflected on the role of subjectivity but also highlighted its contextual underpinnings:

[6] Magalhães, L., Carrasco, C., & Gastaldo, D. (2009).

> *We recognize the indisputable unity between subjectivity and objectivity in the act of knowing. Reality is never just simply the objective datum, the concrete fact, but is also men's perception of it. Once again, this is not a subjectivistic or idealistic affirmation, as it might seem. On the contrary, subjectivism and idealism come into play when the subjective-objective unity is broken.* (Freire, 1985, p. 51)

Nevertheless, I am afraid that we have been unable to understand your words or rather, because they require a great deal of commitment, we might be fearful of them. Could this fear alone explain our hesitation to embrace a social perspective of occupation? There are numerous references to the humanity of fear in your books.

> *The more you recognize your fear as a consequence of your attempt to practice your dream, the more you learn how to put into practice your dream! I never had interviews with the great revolutionaries of the century about their fears!... But all of them felt fear, to the extent that all of them were very faithful to their dreams.* (Shor & Freire, 1987, p. 57)

If I could summarize your arguments, I would say that overcoming fear is to switch our focus to achieving a better understanding of what hope has to do with the historical human enterprise. In his inspiring paper, *Marcuse, Bloch and Freire: reinvigorating a pedagogy of hope*, Van Heertum (2006) remembered you as saying that, 'By returning to his work [Freire], we can recuperate the necessity to look beyond the here and now to the possibility that galvanizes people to act' (p. 46). In order to convey his message, he actually revisited your words: 'For me, history is a time of possibilities, not predeterminations... History is a possibility that we create throughout time, in order to liberate and therefore save ourselves' (Freire, 1998a, as cited by Van Heertum, 2006, p. 47).

I may need to clarify that the reason for my reflections stems from the fact that some themes have been quite absent from the occupational science literature. Differently from your writings, somehow we have been able to *sanitize* our work so that it is free of such contentious topics as *hope* and *love*, for example. I have some hypotheses that may explain it, the main one being that these matters may be considered worthless for an emergent 'scientific' field of study. By the way, there is a very interesting Brazilian philosophy professor, by the name of Viviane Mosé, who mockingly declared that women have not been successful in philosophy because we adopt very pragmatic approaches to philosophical issues. She wrote a beautiful poem suggesting a *Recipe to wash worn out words* (2004, original in Portuguese) in which she claims that some words fade because they are either overused or even misused, while others do not achieve sufficient status to be in such high profile locations as scientific discourse. Her poem always reverberates in my mind when I note the absence of the words love and hope in our occupational science writings. I am then overwhelmed by questions such as: Are we afraid of those words? Are we beyond (or behind) them? Are those words too worn out by overuse and, as a result, are in need of a good, fresh wash? Do we fear that these words (and the concepts behind them) would jeopardize our scientific status? On the other hand, by being so intrinsic to the human experience, shouldn't such themes be an important and inseparable part of the context in which human occupations are performed? I keep asking myself, should we surrender to the urge for specialization and objectivity in order to reach scientific status? Shouldn't we embrace (and celebrate) the fact that the focus of our interests, the occupation and its socio-historical determinants may enable a more innovative synthesis of the connection between body and mind through action, despite its abstract and broad nature? How important is it to engage in praxis in order to establish emancipatory occupations? These are some of the many considerations into which a dialogue with your work may inspire and guide us. I am certain that you could be a great source of wisdom for today's occupational scientists. To be honest, I am hoping that this open letter will engage other researchers in similar conversations with you and your work. As a result, we may be collectively able to contribute to a better understanding of the ways in which it is possible to change the present through announcing/denouncing the future as you have so eloquently emphasized:

> *... though I know that things can get worse, I know that I am able to intervene to improve them ... I am involved with others in making history out of possibility, not simply resigned to fatalistic stagnation ... the future is something to be constructed through trial and error rather than an inexorable vice that determines all our actions.* (Freire, 1998b, p. 34)

The dichotomy between the individual and the social aspects of being is only one example of the potential drawers in which reductionistic thinking may trap us. So, by critically reflecting about such tensions as the artificially crafted tension between the individual and the collective perspectives of occupation, occupational scientists may find a common ground on which we will be able to build a new foundation of knowledge. Eventually, it is hoped that we will be able to advance the discipline while expanding its frontiers.

Professor Freire, my goal with this letter was to begin a dialogue between your writings and some of what I see as the most challenging aspects of this 'new' field of study. I am certain that you will be tolerant in following my erratic paths of reasoning for you have always been very patient with your students. The creation of occupational science has meant a lot for an ever-expanding group of people who are struggling to get it right, despite all the intrinsic uncertainty and uneasiness.

Just returning to your writings has brought me a great deal of hope and comfort. My limitations with the English language prevent me from expressing how proud I am to have had the opportunity to learn from you and to work under your supervision. Within the last 10 years, more than a dozen books have been published in English, which revisited your work. You have been a great source of inspiration to many. Despite language barriers and the difficulties in contextualizing your writings, Brazilians and people from all walks of life across the world have been fighting oppression with the help of your reflections. Hence, your legacy today is more important than ever. As one of Nieto's students wrote in her letter to you, 'May we demonstrate our honor for your work by hearing your voice as we help others find theirs' (Wendy Seger, in Nieto, 2008, p. 65).

Muito obrigada, do fundo do coracao,[7]
With love,

Lilian

[7] Thank you, from the bottom of my heart (in Portuguese).

References

da Silveira, N. (1999). *Cartas a spinoza*. Rio de Janeiro: Francisco Alves.

Facundo, B. (1984). *Freire Inspired Programs in the United States and Puerto Rico: A Critical Evaluation*. Washington, DC: Latino Institute.

Feinberg, W., & Torres, C.A. (2001). Democracy and education: John Dewey and Paulo Freire. In J. Zajda (Ed.), *Education and Society* (3rd ed., pp. 59–70). Melbourne, Australia: James Nicholas Publishers.

Fischman, G., & McLaren, P. (2005). Rethinking critical pedagogy and the Gramscian and Freirean legacies: From organic to committed intellectuals or critical pedagogy, commitment, and praxis. *Cultural Studies ↔ Critical Methodologies*, 5, 425–46. doi: 10.1177/1532708605279701

Freire, P. (n.d.). In *The Ladoc "Keyhole" Series, No. 1* (pp. 3–4). Washington, DC: USCC.

Freire, P. (1972). *Pedagogy of the Oppressed*. New York: Seabury Press.

Freire, P. (1985). *The Politics of Education: Culture, Power and Liberation*. South Hadley, MA: Bergin & Garvey.

Freire, P. (1989). *Education for the Critical Consciousness* (p. 46). New York: Continuum.

Freire, P. (1994). *Pedagogy of Hope*. New York: Continuum.

Freire, P. (1996). *Letters to Cristina: Reflection on My Life and Work*. New York: Routledge.

Freire, P. (1998a). Teachers as cultural workers. Letters to those who dare teach. *The Edge: Critical Studies in Educational Theory* (p. 38). Boulder, CO: Westfield Press.

Freire, P. (1998b). *Pedagogy of Freedom: Ethics, Democracy, and Civic Courage*. Lanham, MD: Rowman & Littlefield.

Furter, P. (1985). Profiles of educators. *Prospects*, **15**, 301–10.

Giroux, H. (2004). Teachers as transformative intellectuals. In A. Canestrari & B. Marlowe (Eds), *Educational Foundations: An Anthology of Critical Readings* (pp. 205–12). Thorofare, NJ: Sage.

Hammell, K.W. (2011). Resisting theoretical imperialism in the disciplines of occupational science and occupational therapy. *British Journal of Occupational Therapy*, 74, 27–33.

Illich, I. (1973). *Deschooling Society*. Harmondsworth: Penguin Books.

Kronenberg, F., Algado, S.S., & Pollard, N. (Eds). (2005). *Occupational Therapy without Borders: Learning from the Spirit of Survivors*. Oxford: Elsevier/Churchill Livingstone.

Kronenberg, F., Pollard, N., & Sakellariou, D. (Eds). (2011). *Occupational Therapy without Borders: Towards an Ecology of Occupation-based Practices* (2nd ed.). Oxford: Churchill Livingstone Elsevier.

Magalhães, L., Carrasco, C., & Gastaldo, D. (2009). Undocumented migrants in Canada: A scoping literature review on health, access to services, and working conditions. *Journal of Immigrant and Minority Health*, **12**, 132–51. doi: 10.1007/s10903-009-9280-5

Mayo, P. (1999). *Gramsci, Freire and Adult Education: Possibilities for Transformative Action*. London: Zed Books.

Mosé, V. (2004). Receita pra Lavar Palavra Suja [Recipe to wash worn out clothes]. Rio de Janeiro, Brazil: Arte Clara.
Nieto, S. (2008). *Dear Paulo: Letters from those who dare teach*. Herndon, VA: Paradigm.
Reid, D. (2011). Mindfulness and flow in occupational engagement: Presence in doing. *Canadian Journal of Occupational Therapy*, 78, 50–6.
Roberts, P. (2000). *Education, Literacy and Humanization: Exploring the Work of Paulo Freire*. London: Bergin & Garvey.
Shor, I., & Freire, P. (1987). *A Pedagogy for Liberation: Dialogues on Transforming Education*. South Hadley, MA: Bergin & Garvey.
Thibeault, R. (2002). Occupation and the rebuilding of civil society: Notes from the war zone. *Journal of Occupational Science*, 9, 38–47.
Townsend, E., & Wilcock, A.A. (2004). Occupational justice and client-centred practice: A dialogue in progress. *Canadian Journal of Occupational Therapy*, 71, 75–87.
Van Heertum, R. (2006). Marcuse, Bloch and Freire: Reinvigorating a pedagogy of hope. *Policy Futures in Education*, 4, 45–51.
Vieira, A. (2008). Cartas pedagógicas. In D. Streck, E. Redin, & J. J. Zitkoski, (Eds) *Dicionário Paulo Freire* (2nd ed., pp. 71–3). Belo Horizonte: Autêntica Editora. [in Portuguese].
Wallerstein, N., & Freudenberg, N. (1998). Linking health promotion and social justice: A rationale and two case stories. *Health Education Research, Theory & Practice*, 13, 451–7.
Whiteford, G. (2000). Occupational deprivation: Global challenge in the new millennium. *British Journal of Occupational Therapy*, 63, 200–4.
Wilcock, A.A. (1998). *An Occupational Perspective of Health*. Thorofare, NJ: Slack.
Yerxa, E.J. (1993). Occupational science: A new source of power for participants in occupational therapy. *Journal of Occupational Science: Australia*, 1, 3–9.
Yerxa, E.J. (2009). Infinite distance between the *I* and the *It*. *American Journal of Occupational Therapy*, 63, 490–7. doi: 10.5014/ajot.63.4.490
Yoo, S.-S. (2007). Freirian legacies in popular education. *Korean Journal of Educational Policy*, 42, 73–94.

Part II
Understanding occupation

3 Transactionalism: Occupational science and the pragmatic attitude

Malcolm P. Cutchin and Virginia A. Dickie

Occupation matters! This is what occupational scientists argue through their descriptions, interpretations, and explanations of occupation in human life. All such arguments are supported, implicitly or explicitly, by some theoretical position(s). The theoretical bases of arguments about occupation also, therefore, matter very much. While strong theory is needed to support the science, occupational scientists want that theory to be nimble enough to handle the complexity of occupation. Moreover, occupational scientists need theory that will enable them to draw sound inferences about occupation that improve upon those that have come before and are relevant to current and future research. However, the choice and use of theory for scholarship has ultimate, and greatest, value as it flows through inquiries and into the lives and communities that occupational scientists intend to improve.

The notion that theory should not only serve science but be evaluated by how it makes a difference in the world is the main concern of the philosophical tradition called pragmatism.[1] Within that tradition there is a strong emphasis on how to theorize action. The concern for what works, that is, how to create a better world, is logically connected to needing to know how action occurs. If scientists and theoreticians want to *make* a better place for themselves and others, they need to know how the previous process of making erred and improve upon it. For occupational scientists, this concern with action is appealing for at least two reasons. First, action

[1] The term 'pragmatism' is problematic in a number of ways, but for the sake of simplicity we will adhere to this most common label for the philosophical approach from which we draw. For more about pragmatism as a loosely defined school of thought and how Dewey's version of it fits, see Shook and Margolis (2009).

Occupational Science: Society, Inclusion, Participation, First Edition.
Edited by Gail Whiteford and Clare Hocking.

is central to understanding occupation itself because all occupations are a form of action (Cutchin *et al.*, 2008). Second, the pragmatic attitude and the corresponding theory of action – what has become known as transactionalism – seem particularly relevant to an occupational science that is concerned with issues that speak to making a better world, such as social justice, inclusion and participation. Transactionalism challenges occupational scientists to think differently about the most central concept of the discipline – occupation – but the broader current of pragmatism, and philosopher John Dewey's version of it in particular, helps to flesh out the wider significance of transactionalism for occupational scientists and therapists.

In this chapter, we begin with an overview of the emergence of transactionalism in occupational science and suggest how it is distinct and why we believe that it adds significant value to the discipline. We then extend the story with more recent contributions to the transactional view of occupation. The second wave of development sets the stage for the addition of more elements drawn from John Dewey's coherent world view. Although the first two waves of work on transactionalism would be enough to suggest its significance for critical perspectives on society, inclusion and participation, we will present additional concepts from Deweyan scholarship that further emphasize the value and potential of this perspective for occupational science. We conclude the chapter by suggesting why transactionalism and a broader Deweyan pragmatic attitude have exciting potential for an occupational science interested in making a difference for individuals and societies.

Transactionalism emerges in occupational science

The emergence of what has been termed the 'transactional' perspective in occupational science is recent, but there is a back-story that helps place the perspective in context. In 1920s America, the new profession of occupational therapy was given credibility as well as additional conceptual basis by the famous physician Adolph Meyer. Influenced by Dewey and other pragmatist philosophers, Meyer presented a paper at the 1921 meeting of the young National Society for the Promotion of Occupational Therapy (Meyer, 1922). He wrote that:

> ... *our conception of man is that of an organism that maintains and balances itself in the world of reality and actuality by being in active life and active use, i.e., using and living and acting its time in harmony with its own nature and the nature about it.* (p. 5)

Meyer also implied that occupational therapy reflected the practice of the new American philosophy of pragmatism in emphasizing the relationship among person, environment and activity, as well as intervening to maximize opportunities to balance the relationship. The importance of these concepts was realized long afterwards, with the development of an understanding of the underlying pragmatic philosophy and what it could mean for occupational science.

In the decades following World War II, John Dewey's philosophical importance waned. However, in disciplines such as philosophy and education, a resurgence of scholarly interest in Dewey's philosophy occurred in the 1980s (Bernstein, 1992) and continues in the present. The scholarship that followed the new interest in Dewey's work was mainly philosophical, but scholars also developed assessments of pragmatism for inquiry in the social sciences (e.g., Emirbayer, 1997; Smith, 1984). As part of that early re-engagement with pragmatism and the special interest in Dewey (the most significant classical pragmatist) Malcolm Cutchin began a series of studies exploring the value of Deweyan pragmatism for theorizing human action in a variety of real-world contexts, such as the integration of rural doctors into their communities and the transition to community care settings by older adults (1997, 1999, 2001, 2003).[2] Cutchin later became engaged professionally with occupational scientists and began to question existing conceptualizations of occupation from a pragmatist perspective. In a subsequent publication, Cutchin (2004) began the argument that would become the start of a continuing discourse about transactionalism in occupational science.

That initial critique of existing theory focused on the problem of 'adaptation-to-the-environment' and posed Dewey's form of pragmatism as an alternative theorization of the relationship between people and their environments. The primary points of the argument suggested that prior thought on the matter had construed the environment as something completely separate from a person – a 'container' in which people existed. In addition to critiquing that dualistic thinking about people and the environment, Cutchin argued that the prevailing view of adaptation suggested action as too subjective and internalized, independent of the relations that actually existed between people and their places of experience. Cutchin's third primary point was that existing theory that attempts to overcome such dualisms and subjectivity, such as the Model of Human Occupation, were too mechanistic, relying on input-output and feedback models in their thinking about how people and environments are related. In contrast to these problems in the theories about adaptation, Cutchin suggested that Dewey's argument for the continuous or non-dualistic (holistic) character of experience was more appropriate to occupational science. Dewey's focus on the 'problematic situation' as a basis for human action and how people 'coordinate' with their environments, most often by restructuring the context rather than personally adapting, was proposed as a more useful theoretical viewpoint. Part of the argument at that stage was that humans' physical, social and cultural milieus are always part of who they are, how they think, and what they do. Consequently, their thinking/acting (e.g., occupation) was suggested as being in continual relationship with the environment.

At the same time that Cutchin was developing his critique of 'adaptation-to-the-environment', Virginia Dickie was studying small-scale craft production and marketing (Dickie, 1996, 1998, 2003a) and contemporary quilt-making (Dickie, 2003b, 2004) from a political economy perspective and finding the existing theory and language of occupational science to be inadequate to support the understanding of occupation she was developing. Likewise, Ruth Humphry was observing the profoundly social and contextualized nature of the way very young children learned occupations, which could not be accounted for by theories that located development within the child (Humphry, 2005). Following on the heels of Cutchin's initial proposal, Dickie, Cutchin, and Humphry (2006) argued for Deweyan philosophy to undergird thought

[2] Among others influential in Cutchin's work is the pragmatist Jim Garrison, who was invited as a keynote speaker for the 2001 AOTF-sponsored conference on habit and who published an important article on Dewey's philosophy and occupational therapy (Garrison, 2002).

in occupational science about occupation *per se*. Their article presented more specifics about the theory of transactionalism. The rationale for their argument was a critique of occupational science's implicit and explicit use of individualism (focus on independent, subjective individuals) and the concomitant use of dualistic thinking about people as apart from their environments. Although this critique had been lodged earlier by Hocking (2000), Dickie *et al.* extended the argument and directed attention to the limitations of such a view in cutting out the multiple and complex influences on occupation that work together with individual action. The authors claimed that 'an understanding of individual experience is a necessary but *insufficient* condition for understanding occupation that occurs through complex contexts' (Dickie *et al.*, p. 83). The problem of the individualistic occupation perspective, they explained, was that of tearing asunder the holism of occupations and narrowing the focus on individual subjectivity with the resulting loss of the richness and complexity of occupations. The proposed solution was the theoretical perspective of transactionalism.

While Dickie *et al.* (2006) particularly looked at the language of early occupational science theoretical literature, they were also concerned with an emphasis on individual meaning in many research articles. Earlier, Dickie (2003b) raised the question 'If, instead of studying "the human as an occupational being" [Yerxa, 1993], we were to study occupation as a human enterprise, would our discoveries be different?' (p. 121). In other words, she was calling for a shift in focus away from how occupation was experienced by individuals, in and of themselves, to study that encompassed the totality of occupation as part of context. There have been a number of studies in the occupational science literature that have taken this approach, for example Riley's study of a weaving guild (2008), and Asaba's study of a group in a mental health setting that engaged in what he termed an 'assembly occupation' (2008). These two studies included cultural and historical dimensions as well as individual meanings. International cross-cultural research focused on the holiday food preparation of older women in Thailand, New Zealand and Kentucky incorporated elements beyond, but linked to, individual experience and meaning such as culture, tradition, seasonal weather, objects, place and change over time (Hocking, Wright-St. Clair, & Bunrayong, 2002; Shordike & Pierce, 2005; Wright-St. Clair *et al.*, 2004). Russell's 2008 literature-based study of the phenomenon of 'tagging' maps out the long history of graffiti, the personal and social meanings of tagging among those who practice the activity as well as the physical and legal risks they assume in doing so, the effect of tagging on the larger community, and both destructive and constructive possibilities arising from tagging. These studies demonstrate the potential of holistic approaches to building knowledge of occupation.

A focus on individual experiences and meanings has been prominent in the occupational science literature, however, even in studies of group occupations. For example, Tonneijck, Kinébanian and Josephsson (2008) studied singing in a choir from the perspectives of those they interviewed, and focused their findings on their participants' individual experiences within the choral setting. Likewise, Jacob, Guptill and Sumsion (2009) addressed the individual experiences of nine members of a university choir, gathering data through interviews and developing findings that were individually focused. In contrast, Womack (2009) completed an ethnographic study of a women's chorus in which she looked at the chorus as a whole, situated across time and place and embedded in social and political concerns of the day. The occupation of singing in a chorus was one of many occupations that created and sustained the chorus over 25 years.

In order to formulate a theoretical basis for a more contextualized view of occupation, Dickie *et al.* (2006) used work by Dewey and Bentley (1949)[3] and later pragmatists such as Garrison (2001) to propose that the holistic view of people acting in the world (or 'organism-in-the-environment-as-a-whole' as Dewey and Bentley put it) was of greater advantage to occupational scientists than an individualistic perspective. Transactionalism suggests that neither self-action nor interaction provide sufficient understanding of the way in which people and their environments co-define and co-constitute each other (Sullivan, 2001). An additional point that Garrison (2001) emphasized is essential: Dewey's position about the continuity of any environment and individual is that they are continually related by the necessity of 'functional coordination'. If people are to function and to maximize function – and occupation is a particularly relevant example – it is not just a person acting independently of an environment; there must be constant coordination of the relationship between the environment and person. Often this active coordination is very subtle and unrealized, such as the way most people walk up a flight of stairs without any conscious consideration of the height, depth and surface of the stairs, but even such taken-for-granted functional coordination sometimes requires substantial change, as for example, when people climb the stairs with their arms full, or develop techniques for managing stairs after a leg injury. But functional coordination can be a response to major environmental threats. For example, determining how and acting to rebuild a home collapsed in an earthquake, with few resources and reliance on the help of far-flung charitable agencies, also is a type of functional coordination.

Whether subtle or obvious and substantial, functional coordination as such is viewed as a 'transaction' via the dynamic, coordinated restructuring of relationships of person and situation. It is this focus on action inherent in the relationships among things (e.g., people and aspects of their environment), and action as those relationships are modified in any way, that makes transactionalism a *relational* theory. In other words, it is the relations among things, not what takes place within things, which should hold a scientist's attention. The old adage 'it takes two to tango' is perhaps descriptive enough to get the point across: a tango dancer cannot dance without a partner (or particular music, or the ongoing history of that dance form) just as individuals cannot act without coordinating functionally with their current situations. It is this action and its ongoing redirection, reshaping and reemphasis that keeps the whole as well as the parts functional. In short, it is the way in which people inhabit their worlds.

For occupational science, a transactional perspective can support knowledge development and translational research targeted toward entities such as political systems, populations and environmental concerns at the same time that it problematizes concepts and theories of occupation that do not account for more than the

[3] We believe it is important to note here that while some see this very late work of Dewey as being too influenced by Bentley and too extreme in its naturalism and technical logic (e.g., Jackson, 2009), others point to the fact that the main tenants of the transactional view posited in this late book were expressed early and throughout much of Dewey's career and were consistent with his brand of humanistic and socially oriented philosophy (Thayer & Thayer, 1978). As Garrison (2001) and Alexander (2009) have argued, the transactional perspective was already developed in Dewey's classic critique of the reflex arc concept in psychology (Dewey, 1896/1998b).

individual actor. Laliberte Rudman's (2005) analysis of the newspaper constructions of retirement provides an example of how some emerging research into contextual aspects of occupation is moving in the same direction as a transactional perspective. Using a critical discourse analysis approach, Rudman identified four 'ideal retiree subjectivity types' which were constructed through writings in a major Canadian newspaper and linked these types to the 'neoliberal technologies of government' (2005, p. 156). She went on to point out how these discourses promote certain occupations while neglecting or degrading others. In a later paper, Laliberte Rudman (2010) presented the construct of 'occupational possibilities', examined within the framework of governmentality, and positioned this theoretical work within the study of the situated nature of occupation. We view the transactional perspective as additionally supportive of, and generally consistent with, Laliberte Rudman's approach in that it offers a way to understand relational dynamics between contextual elements and people in situations.

The first attempts we made to redirect occupational science theory toward the holistic and relational theory of Dewey's pragmatism were noteworthy in that they offered both a critique of other theoretical orientations as well as a different way forward. Occupational scientists were asked to examine occupation with a much broader perspective, and given theory and language that supported intellectual and practice engagement with population, political, environmental and economic issues. Yet the argument at that point was incomplete (and as will become evident, it remains so). In the next section, we aim to review additional components of the case for transactionalism in occupational science that subsequently have engaged our thinking.

Further development of transactionalism

The argument for transaction is difficult to understand in and of itself. The points about continuity, holism, the centrality of the environment (social and otherwise), functional coordination and relationship of elements in a situation, and action being located in the relationships and their coordination, are logically connected but do not lend themselves well to graphic representation. Furthermore the argument asks occupational scientists to shift from dominant views about occupation – as it has come to be understood via other theoretical perspectives. As important, however, is the need to expand the theory to suggest how occupation, as a fundamental form of transaction, is understood to happen. In addition, a better grasp of how environments and people are related and how that influences action is needed. Moreover, transactionalism shares certain aspects with other theories of interest in occupational science, notably complexity science (Eakman, 2007; Fogelberg & Frauwirth, 2010; Gray, Kennedy, & Zemke, 1996; Gray & Zemke, 1996), phenomenology (Barber, 2004, 2006; Gray, 1997), and other theories of action (Strauss, as cited by Hocking, 2000). The similarities and the differences between transactionalism and these other perspectives, including issues of fit with occupational science, need further investigation.

A second set of publications by occupational scientists has begun to address those issues. Cutchin *et al.* (2008) conducted a more careful reading of Deweyan literature in an attempt to deepen the understanding of action, and thereby, what a transactional view of occupation means. The authors focused on three dimensions of action that are essential to Dewey's understanding: habit, context and creativity.

Habit was central to Dewey's action theory and is thus important to any transactional understanding of occupation. Dewey (1922/1957) stated that habits are 'acquired predispositions to *ways* or modes of response' (p. 40). In this sense, habits are often below the level of consciousness, generating thoughts and actions without effort on the part of the individual.[4] What Cutchin *et al.* (2008) disclosed, however, is that Dewey's argument about the source and use of habits in action – and for our purposes, in occupation – went much beyond that statement. Dewey argued persuasively that habits arise from *engagement* in social activities, and Cutchin (2007) posited that this included not only the 'social customs' that Dewey noted as formative of habits but also the physical and symbolic landscapes of that encourage habits of thought and doing. In addition, Dewey suggested that people gain many habits that work together in 'configurations', specifically assembled for the particular situation, that enable thought, movement, and any other form of action. Indeed, any functional coordination at the heart of a transaction has at its core a unique configuration of habits, assembled and related to the ongoing action of a situation. The more habits people have at their disposal, the more potential they have to employ different habit configurations in relation to a situation and in response to changes in the situation. According to Dewey, habits come from participation in the world and exist only in the relationship that creates, supports or limits the functionality of the habit as it is configured with many others to enable action. Thus habits can never be viewed as internal to the individual. This is of profound importance for thinking about occupation and social change. Any circumstance that restricts participation (such as job discrimination based on one's real or assumed immigration status, keeping children indoors because their neighbourhoods are unsafe, imprisonment without opportunities for work and education, extended illness and extended dwelling in refugee camps) decreases the possibilities for those who are restricted to develop and use functional habits.

Consider, for example, people who become unemployed because their employers relocate their jobs to areas with lower labour costs. Over time, they are restricted from participating in many community and home activities because of lack of funds (and social stigma related to not working). Without these avenues of participation, people may resort to narrow ranges of relatively non-functional habits such as staying at home, not bothering to clean the house, and avoiding places where they might see people who know them from their working days (Aldrich & Callanan, 2011). In this way, political and economic factors (and actors) may create circumstances where individuals develop habits that tend to restrict their social worlds.

As Cutchin (2007) and Cutchin *et al.* (2008) proposed, habit becomes the basis of all action, and for that matter, all occupation. The point is not that people are automatons with a pre-programmed set of habits to use, however. The *context* of action, what Dewey termed the *situation*, is always part of the *process* of action. Situations and/or

[4] From Dewey's point of view, thought is a subset of action and should not be considered especially distinct from other forms of action. In other words, as the rest of the evolving argument suggests, thought occurs only in concert with the world through which we live; it is never to be considered internal and separate from that world.

people's relationship to them change, and even if relatively stable for the moment, set the stage for the possibilities of action. As such, Dewey argued that situations are generative of action. He wrote that 'a situation is a whole in virtue of its immediately pervasive quality... the situation as a qualitative whole is sensed or felt' (Dewey, 1938/1998a, p. 384). He added that 'a qualitative and qualifying situation is present as the background and the control of every experience' (Dewey, 1938/1998a, p. 385). Because situations are qualitatively singular – individual in their own right – they at some point require people to inquire (investigate, reflect) about what to do with them and about how to functionally re-coordinate with them (and to what ends). There are always multiple possibilities, some of which people do not know until they inquire into them (i.e., try them out either in reality or in their imaginations). This requires creativity and is why humans, with their habit configurations, are more than automatons. A logical conclusion, therefore, is that occupational scientists should incorporate the situation as part of any study of occupational experiences.

In determining the nature of possible transactions, including occupations, a person is required to assess the qualities of the situation and what, if anything, needs to change in order to feel balance, or as Dewey often called it, 'harmony'. As Cutchin *et al.* (2008) discussed (drawing on Fesmire, 2003), this call to deliberation means one has to both draw on an existing stock of habits (thoughts/actions) as a form of 'intelligence' and on 'imagination'. Imagination in this sense is the ability to see possible new situational arrangements in light of the current situation. People develop multiple images of what might be, by developing different novel habit configurations, and then use their moral sensibilities – another product of social customs and experience in different situations (Cutchin, 2007) – to determine the best course of action to coordinate. Dewey went so far as to suggest that people enter into a dramatic rehearsal of these possibilities to determine which might be best (Fesmire, 2003). This process of ongoing action within the stream of experience in different situations was, for Dewey, always a process of inquiry. As we will explain in the next section, however, this transactive process is not an individual affair (in contrast to a phenomenological perspective). In Dewey's philosophic system, he urged one to recall the role of *the social* in the process.

In addition to breaking down the transactive process into component subprocesses, in order to enhance the understanding of action and occupations as transactional, other recent efforts have taken a step back in order to think more broadly about transactionalism and Dewey's broader philosophy vis-à-vis other theoretical systems. Aldrich (2008) developed a careful comparison of complexity theory and Dewey's transactionalism as they have been used in occupational science. She concluded that while there is some overlap in the two theoretical perspectives, transactionalism's antidualistic (holistic) foundation provides a major advantage over complexity theory. Among other characteristics that Aldrich suggested as providing transactionalism with an edge in the comparison are its focus on uncertainty in the world, more organic (less mechanical) language, and its attention to the 'socially funded, relational nature of experience [which] helps guard it against concerns about applicability in non-Western cultures' (p. 154).

Cutchin and his colleagues (Cutchin, 2008; Cutchin, Dickie, & Humphry, 2006) have also compared Deweyan philosophy to theoretical approaches that are of interest to occupational science. They suggested that phenomenological theory and Dewey's work shared some important aspects but that the individual intentionality and meaning that is at the core of phenomenological thought does not go far enough toward describing experience. In a Deweyan view, the problematic material transactions of ongoing life that develop as part of indeterminate situations create reflective action and thereby, meaning (but this action and meaning-making are taking place with all of the participants in the situation). Cutchin (2008) argued that social constructionist philosophies, such as those viewed as structural, post-structural and post-modern thought, have more in common with Deweyan meta-theory than phenomenology. Yet, he concluded that based on analyses by a number of philosophers, Dewey stood apart from other social constructionists through his theory of transaction.

The broader scope of the Deweyan pragmatic attitude

Dewey's primary concern in developing his philosophy was to give a better understanding of human experience, but that understanding was developed in order to improve civilization by enrichment of individual citizens and their abilities to engage in social life (Jackson, 2009; Putnam, 2009). His attempt at a reconstruction of philosophy to focus on experience suggested many elements, including an argument for 'criticism' as a tool for the reconstruction of social goods; that is, how we should go about valuing aspects of society and changing them in response to the results of that valuing. Related to valuing, Dewey also emphasized ethics in the analysis of action; moral concerns were to be placed squarely in the middle of an assessment of real-world activities.[5] His concern for criticism and moral elements of daily life are associated with another key motif in his writing: enriching people and their lives through 'growth'. For Dewey, growth implied 'the continuing flowering and actualization of possibilities ... the actual enhancement of an individual's life... and the development of new powers of action' (Boisvert, 1998, p. 59). Through these and other concepts, Dewey wanted to reconstruct the philosophical tradition so that it would discard the dualisms that it had used to paint itself into an intellectual corner and to deal with life as it is experienced in the full sense of embodied, emotional and emplaced living. Moreover, he wanted people to have the tools to reconstruct their situations, their customs, their institutions, and thereby improve their lives. Dewey's philosophy provides a set of conceptual tools – what he called a 'metaphysical ground-map' – for this purpose. This 'pragmatic attitude' espoused by Dewey was one in which people could make a better world for those in it now and for those yet to come. That attitude has certain traits that also need to be outlined.

Dewey's metaphysics indicates a 'denotive method' where people experience qualitative wholes, attend to particular traits of those wholes, assign symbolic significances to those traits, develop values and judgements about the situation, and use those judgements to act (test) and change the situation (when it is deemed necessary to do so).[6] The map metaphor represents people's selection and symbolization of the significances in the situation. The metaphor is useful, because as with

[5] Particularly good sources for more insight into these emphases in Dewey's pragmatic attitude are Gouinlock (1972) and Dewey (1922/1957).

[6] We draw on the insightful work of Garrison (2005) in this section on the metaphysical ground-map.

geographical maps, Dewey's metaphysical map is provisional (based on the fallibility of current knowledge) and skewed by human interests; pluralism and change mean it is uncertain and unfinished. As such, the ground-map is a working theory. In addition, the metaphysical map is a tool for inquiry and criticism. It allows people to view differences and meanings, but it also offers a way to value (desire) goods (aspects of the world that support or enhance life) in the world and to try and enact or create them through judgements about how to successfully do so. In other ways, the map denotes a set of transactions of person and world, experience and judgements. The metaphysical map is transformational because it generates values and criticism, and because it suggests inquiry and transactional change through a situation. The map represents occupation because it suggests all the basics of action on which all occupation rests, and it goes the next step by suggesting how one can improve occupation and well-being. In a final sense, Dewey's metaphysical map is scientific, but it is science as art. It allows imagination and creativity in action and occupation. Its qualitative basis means that humans must use sensing and interpretation, communication and narration for growth – personal and social. The power of Dewey's metaphysical ground-map is discursive – it is not in the map itself; rather, the map's power resides in a person's transaction with it and the vision and actions taken through its use. Those visions and actions are always related to experience, and as with the map itself, are contingent and reconstructable because Dewey 'believes that we are active participants in an unfinished and unfinishable universe' (Garrison, 2005, p. 835).

It is at this point that we can begin to make more concrete sense of the value of Dewey's theoretical perspective for understanding occupation as well as inclusion, participation and social change. If we are all participants in an unfinished universe, how should we best participate and to what ends? The Dewey scholar Raymond Boisvert (1998) noted that Dewey's pragmatic attitude:

> ... *culminates quite reasonably in the challenge of responsible involvement: the call to participate in channeling the energies of our surrounding world in such a way as to preserve and enhance the goods we already have, while attempting to secure new ones.* (p. 26)

For Dewey, the basis of involvement and participation was community.[7] Community is essential 'because it makes possible a more diversified and enriching life for all members' (Campbell, 1995, p. 172). Maximal participation in community life not only enhances individuality and growth of persons through their specific contributions, but it extends those benefits throughout the community through communication and the development of shared values and habits (Boisvert, 1998; Campbell, 1995). Participation in community – and occupation is a main mode of participation in any community – is for Dewey the primary way humans grow their capacities, as individuals and societies. And it is through that concern for social improvement (or meliorism, as Dewey frequently called it) as well as individual flowering (for the

[7] Campbell (1995, pp. 172–3) discussed the various meanings of community for Dewey. While he sometimes used community more generally to denote any type of group or association, he also used a more restrictive sense of 'a public' engaged in the democratic process of maintaining the place, institutions and associated affairs that supports its members. We prefer the latter sense to be considered the primary one here.

two go hand-in-hand in a transactional relationship) that Dewey's pragmatic attitude may best be described in the word 'responsibility.' As Boisvert (1998) put it:

> *For Dewey, humans are participants in a world of ongoing, interwoven, contingent affairs. It is incumbent upon them to act in such a way that will encourage the realization of those possibilities appropriate to flourishing sociopolitical life. Such a life can be realized in no other way.* (p. 26)

And Dewey's (1922/1957) sense of responsibility was even more ambitious than that.

> *The best we can accomplish for posterity is to transmit unimpaired and with some increment of meaning the environment that makes it possible to maintain the habits of decent and refined life. Our individual habits are links in forming the endless chain of humanity. Their significance depends upon the environment inherited from our forerunners, and it is enhanced as we foresee the fruits of our labors in the world in which our successors live.* (p. 23)

As occupational scientists, we see occupation as a central part of acting in ways that will help reach these lofty ideals. In the next section, we turn to a concluding assessment of the implications for occupational science of transactionalism and the pragmatic attitude of John Dewey. His ground-map is there for us to use, but it is up to us to determine the best ways to put it to work.

Conclusion: Implications for occupational science

The editors of this book argue for a discipline of occupational science that is relevant to global occupational realities such as poverty, lack of education, environmental degradation, participation in antisocial occupations, and other social and economic conditions that are affected by and affect occupations. A theoretical perspective that focuses on individualism is inadequate to support such a science, and because we support the editors' argument, we see a great need for theories that will ground the thinking and research of occupational science in a broader view that suits those ambitious aims. While we think there is much in Dewey's transactionalism that is commensurate with such a task, we admit that there are always other theoretical alternatives. Moreover, Dewey developed his thinking in a particular time and place, which raises questions of currency and relevance. Would transactionalism and the corresponding pragmatic attitude be relevant to occupation in cultures throughout the world? Does a philosophy that came to prominence in the early twentieth century pertain to problems in the early twenty-first century? Boisvert (1998) concluded the answer was yes because Dewey's philosophy and pragmatic attitude provide a schema for 'thinking our own time' (p. 158). We hasten to suggest that the schema also applies to different places and cultures. But will transactionalism and the pragmatic attitude work as a basis for theorizing and engaging with the problems occupational science is tackling, including the important ones behind the development of this book? Ultimately, that question will be answered only by the research produced by occupational scientists themselves. We are optimistic about the potential and outcomes.

The pragmatic attitude derived from Dewey is one made up of key metaphors that are helpful in addressing the question. Among those metaphors, 'inquiry', 'community' and 'responsibility' allow the pragmatic attitude to add significant value to the core theory of transactionalism. Dewey's pragmatism suggests a process, or method, for engaging with the world – whether as a scientist or not. That engagement is twofold, with a concern for the sufficient conduct of everyday life as well as the growth of people and communities through change that enhances the common good. In either case, the process is always a type of shared inquiry in which communities are involved through their influence on members, and the implications that members' actions hold for communities. People therefore have a responsibility to others in the community and to the community's well-being as a whole. Others and the community always become a part of inquiry. The point is this: occupational scientists must endeavour to include communal or social problems in the frame of their inquiries. If occupations matter, then the community – however it is defined – matters as well. The pragmatic attitude means that a concern for social justice, inclusion and participation can never truly be separated from the study of occupation.

One concern at this point is that Dewey's perspective focused so much on individuals and communities. It would be easy to frame our argument in these terms alone, but this does not go far enough to address the concerns of occupational science. The pragmatic attitude also allows for consideration of the non-human, however. Voltaire, through Candide (1759/1975), reminded the world that it needs to *cultivate* its gardens, and in doing so he implied fertile earth, seeds, tools, sun and rain, as well as the physical capacities needed by those who do that tending. All of this makes up the dynamic, transactional situation (as do the neighbour's goats or forest deer that are threats to the success of the garden). In that situation people engage in habits developed over time, and work in anticipation of the results they hope to attain. The relative importance of that garden to whether or not one's family eats depends upon many factors beyond the gardener's control (e.g., the opportunities for waged work). All of this, and more, is part of the transactional nature of the occupation of gardening.

The metaphors of the pragmatic attitude provide both a logic and a sentiment for situating occupation as part of larger contextual dynamics. Transaction provides the conceptual power to analyse occupation as the functional coordination of person and situation in order to bring people into greater harmony with their worlds – and to improve well-being. And while a turn to transactionalism provokes by asking occupational scientists to examine and perhaps change their world view about occupation, we believe the provocative request is worth earnest consideration. How occupational scientists decide to go about the particulars of inquiry with the attitude and theory are still emerging and somewhat unknown. We hope the occupational scientists willing to heed the theoretical request can play an important part as participants in an unfinished universe, who work with a pragmatic attitude, and who become engaged in the betterment of various people and communities who struggle for social justice, inclusion, participation and environmental stewardship.

References

Aldrich, R.M. (2008). From complexity theory to transactionalism: Moving occupational science forward in theorizing the complexities of behavior. *Journal of Occupational Science*, **15**, 147–56.

Aldrich, R.M., & Callanan, Y. (2011). Insights about researching discouraged workers. *Journal of Occupational Science*, **18**, 153–66.

Alexander, T.M. (2009). Dewey, dualism, and naturalism. In J.R. Shook & J. Margolis (Eds), *A Companion to Pragmatism* (pp. 184–92). Chichester: John Wiley & Sons, Ltd.

Asaba, E. (2008). Hashi-ire: Where occupation, chopsticks, and mental health intersect. *Journal of Occupational Science*, **15**, 74–9.

Barber, M. (2004). Occupational science and phenomenology: Human activity, narrative and ethical responsibility. *Journal of Occupational Science*, **11**, 105–14.

Barber, M. (2006). Occupational science and the first-person perspective. *Journal of Occupational Science*, **13**, 94–6.

Bernstein, R.J. (1992). The resurgence of pragmatism. *Social Research*, **59**, 813–41.

Boisvert, R. (1998). *John Dewey: Rethinking our Time*. Albany, NY: State University of New York Press.

Campbell, J. (1995). *Understanding John Dewey: Nature and cooperative intelligence*. Chicago: Open Court.

Cutchin, M.P. (1997). Physician retention in rural communities: The perspective of experiential place integration. *Health & Place*, **3**, 25–41.

Cutchin, M.P. (1999). Qualitative explorations in health geography: Using pragmatism and related concepts as guides. *The Professional Geographer*, **51**, 265–74.

Cutchin, M.P. (2001). Deweyan integration: Moving beyond place attachment in elderly migration theory. *International Journal of Aging and Human Development*, **52**, 29–44.

Cutchin, M.P. (2003). The process of mediated aging-in-place: A theoretically and empirically based model. *Social Science and Medicine*, **57**, 1077–90.

Cutchin, M.P. (2004). Using Deweyan philosophy to rename and reframe adaptation-to-environment. *American Journal of Occupational Therapy*, **58**, 303–12.

Cutchin, M.P. (2007). From society to self (and back) through place: Habit in transactional context. *OTJR: Occupation, Participation, and Health*, **27**, 50S–59S.

Cutchin, M.P. (2008). John Dewey's metaphysical ground-map and its implications for geographical inquiry. *Geoforum*, **39**, 1555–65.

Cutchin, M.P., Dickie, V., & Humphry, R. (2006). Transaction versus interpretation, or transaction and interpretation? A response to Michael Barber. *Journal of Occupational Science*, **13**, 97–99.

Cutchin, M.P., Aldrich, R.M., Bailliard, A., & Coppola, S. (2008). Action theories for occupational science: The contributions of Dewey and Bourdieu. *Journal of Occupational Science*, **15**, 157–65.

Dewey, J. (1957). *Human Nature and Conduct: An Introduction to Social Psychology*. New York: The Modern Library. [Originally published in 1922]

Dewey, J. (1998a). Common sense and scientific inquiry (from *Logic: The theory of inquiry*) In L. Hickman & T. Alexander (Eds), *The Essential Dewey, Vol. 1* (pp. 380–90). Bloomington, IN: Indiana University Press. [Original work published in 1938]

Dewey, J. (1998b). The reflex arc concept in psychology. In L. Hickman & T. Alexander (Eds), *The Essential Dewey, Vol.* 2 (pp. 3–18). Bloomington, IN: Indiana University Press [Original work published in 1896]

Dewey, J., & Bentley, A. (1949). *Knowing and the Known*. Boston: Beacon Press.

Dickie, V. (1996). Craft production in Detroit: Spatial, temporal, and social relations of work in the home. *Journal of Occupational Science: Australia*, **3**, 65–71.

Dickie, V. (1998). Households, multiple livelihoods, and the informal economy: A study of American crafters. *Scandinavian Journal of Occupational Therapy*, **5**, 109–18.

Dickie, V. (2003a). Establishing worker identity: A study of people in craftwork. *American Journal of Occupational Therapy*, **57**, 250–61.

Dickie, V. (2003b). The role of learning in quilt making. *Journal of Occupational Science*, **10**, 120–9.

Dickie, V. (2004). From drunkard's path to Kansas cyclones: Discovering creativity inside the blocks. *Journal of Occupational Science*, **11**, 51–7.

Dickie, V., Cutchin, M.P., & Humphry, R. (2006). Occupation as transactional experience: A critique of individualism in occupational science. *Journal of Occupational Science*, **13**, 83–93.

Eakman, A. (2007). Occupation and social complexity. *Journal of Occupational Science*, **14**, 82–91.

Emirbayer, M. (1997). Manifesto for a relational sociology. *American Journal of Sociology*, **103**, 281–317.

Fesmire, S. (2003). *John Dewey and Moral Imagination: Pragmatism in Ethics*. Bloomington, IN: Indiana University Press.

Fogelberg, D., & Frauwirth, S. (2010). A complexity science approach to occupation: Moving beyond the individual. *Journal of Occupational Science*, **17**, 131–9.

Garrison, J. (2001). An introduction to Dewey's theory of functional "trans-action": An alternative paradigm for activity theory. *Mind, Culture, and Activity*, **8**, 275–96.

Garrison, J. (2002). Habits as social tools in context. *Occupational Therapy Journal of Research*, **22**, 11S–17S.

Garrison, J. (2005). Dewey on metaphysics, meaning making, and maps. *Transactions of the Charles S. Peirce Society*, **41**, 818–44.

Gouinlock, J. (1972). *John Dewey's Philosophy of Value*. New York: Humanities Press.

Gray, J. (1997). Application of the phenomenological method to the concept of occupation. *Journal of Occupational Science*, **4**, 5–17.

Gray, J., & Zemke, R. (1996). Dynamic systems theory: An overview. In R. Zemke & F. Clark (Eds), *Occupational Science: The Evolving Discipline* (pp. 297–308). Philadelphia: F.A. Davis.

Gray, J., Kennedy, B., & Zemke, R. (1996). Application of dynamic system theory to occupation. In R. Zemke & F. Clark (Eds), *Occupational Science: The Evolving Discipline* (pp. 309–24). Philadelphia: F.A. Davis.

Hocking, C. (2000). Occupational science: A stock take of accumulated insights. *Journal of Occupational Science*, **7**, 58–67.

Hocking, C., Wright-St. Clair, V., & Bunrayong, W. (2002). The meaning of cooking and recipe work for older Thai and New Zealand women. *Journal of Occupational Science*, **9**, 117–27.

Humphry, R. (2005). Model of processes transforming occupations: Exploring societal and social influences. *Journal of Occupational Science*, **12**, 27–35.

Jackson, P.W. (2009). John Dewey. In J.R. Shook & J. Margolis (Eds), *A Companion to Pragmatism* (pp. 54–66). Chichester: John Wiley & Sons, Ltd.

Jacob, C., Guptill, C., & Sumsion, T. (2009). Motivation for continuing involvement in a leisure-based choir: The lived experiences of university choir members. *Journal of Occupational Science*, **16**, 187–93.

Laliberte Rudman, D. (2005). Understanding political influences on occupational possibilities: An analysis of newspaper constructions of retirement. *Journal of Occupational Science*, **12**, 149–60.

Laliberte Rudman, D. (2010). Occupational possibilities. *Journal of Occupational Science*, **17**, 55–9.

Meyer, A. (1922). The philosophy of occupation therapy. *Archives of Occupational Therapy*, **1**, 1–10.

Putnam, R.A. (2009). Democracy and value inquiry. In J.R. Shook & J. Margolis (Eds), *A Companion to Pragmatism* (pp. 278–89). Chichester: John Wiley & Sons, Ltd.

Riley, J. (2008). Weaving an enhanced sense of self and a collective sense of self through creative textile-making. *Journal of Occupational Science*, **15**, 63–73.

Shook, J.R., & Margolis, J. (Eds). (2009). *A Companion to Pragmatism*. Chichester: John Wiley & Sons, Ltd.

Shordike, A., & Pierce, D. (2005). Cooking up Christmas in Kentucky: Occupation and tradition in the stream of time. *Journal of Occupational Science*, **12**, 140–8.

Smith, S.J. (1984). Practicing humanistic geography. *Annals of the Association of American Geographers*, **70**, 207–25.

Sullivan, S. (2001). *Living Across and Through Skins: Transactional Bodies, Pragmatism and Feminism*. Bloomington, IN: Indiana University Press.

Thayer, H., & Thayer, V. (1978). Introduction. In J. Boydston (Ed.), *John Dewey: The Middle Works, Vol. 6, How We Think, and Selected Essays 1910–1911* (pp. ix–xxviii). Carbondale & Edwardsville, IL: Southern Illinois University Press.

Tonneijck, H., Kinébanian, A., & Josephsson, S. (2008). An exploration of choir singing: Achieving wholeness through challenge. *Journal of Occupational Science*, **15**, 173–80.

Voltaire, J.(1975). *Candide*. New York: Random House. [Original work published 1759]

Womack, J. (2009). *Singing for Our Lives: Exploring the Interaction of Community, Feminism and Musical Performance in the Common Woman Chorus*. Unpublished master's thesis, University of North Carolina at Chapel Hill (Folklore). Retrieved from http://dc.lib.unc.edu/cdm4/item_viewer.php?CISOROOT=/etd&CISOPTR=2595 (last accessed 12 June 2011)

Wright-St Clair, V., Bunrayong, W., Vittayakorn, S., Rattakorn, P., & Hocking, C. (2004). Offerings: Food traditions of older Thai women at Songkran. *Journal of Occupational Science*, **11**, 115–24.

4 Understanding the discursive development of occupation: Historico-political perspectives

Sarah Kantartzis and Matthew Molineux

Occupational science emerged in the late twentieth century in the English-speaking academic world of the United States (USA), and spread rapidly to institutions in Australia, Canada, Japan, New Zealand and the United Kingdom (Laliberte Rudman *et al.*, 2008), the majority also being anglophone. The expressed purpose of this new science was the study of human occupation in all its forms, functions and meanings (Yerxa *et al.*, 1990), to expand the existing understanding of occupation in the therapeutic context of occupational therapy.

Occupational science, like other academic disciplines and professions, had its genesis within a particular society, at a particular place and time. Foucault has drawn attention to the importance of understanding the broader conditions of possibility within which a formal body of knowledge emerges (Scheurich & McKenzie, 2005). For occupational scientists, this means acknowledging that their understandings of occupation reflected their own experiences and knowledge of daily life in their social world; that is, their understandings were coherent with their experience of reality. For occupational science, understanding of the contextual influences entails exploring the complex context of practices, relations, meanings and norms related to daily life and of activity in particular, which existed in the USA in the second half of the twentieth century.

The conditions of possibility of occupational science also included the existing knowledge and experience of occupation held within occupational therapy, as one of the stated forces leading to its development was a need for that profession to re-discover its roots; its focus on occupation (Wilcock, 2001; Yerxa, 1993). Emerging more than 50 years after the profession was founded, also in the USA, occupational

Occupational Science: Society, Inclusion, Participation, First Edition.
Edited by Gail Whiteford and Clare Hocking.

science explicitly took on the values and traditions expressed by the founders of occupational therapy and later writers who focused on the importance of occupation (Yerxa *et al.*, 1990).

It is therefore important to consider the degree to which current understandings of occupation are dominated by a Western, anglophone, and middle-class view of reality. This need exists despite earlier calls to increase awareness of issues of power and the need to embrace diversity and situatedness in the current era of post-modernism (Whiteford, Townsend, & Hocking, 2000), because these have not been addressed in relation to the nature and characteristics of the concept of occupation itself.

Following a brief discussion of the construction of the social world, the influence of institutions related to belief, governance, education and economy on everyday activity will be explored. We argue that dominant Western social institutions such as the Protestant church, capitalism and industrialization, democracy and character-based education have had multiple influences on both the form of occupation and related beliefs and values. The influence of this discourse on the conceptualization of occupation found in the occupational science literature will be explored. Understandings reached during a study of the daily life and occupations of the inhabitants of a small Greek town will be drawn on to provide a contrasting view of occupation from a different historico-political perspective. We argue that critique of the dominant Western discourse is essential if occupation is to be understood within other social groups and in other parts of the world.

The nature of reality

Characteristic of the post-modern era is an understanding of the contextualized and diverse nature of knowledge (Whiteford *et al.*, 2000). It is understood that social reality is constructed (Berger & Luckman, 1966), and that an individual's world view exerts a powerful influence on how he or she experiences and interprets events (Cobern, 1993). Post-modern theories discuss the nature of the embodied and situated knowledge of the particular world in which an individual is brought up (Bourdieu, 1977), and how individuals' actions are both enabled and constrained by the social structures which these actions produce and reproduce, as structure and agency shape each other (Archer, 2000; Giddens, 1984). These theories emphasize how individuals' experiences of the world around them, their possibilities for action, and the values and meanings that they give to these actions are linked to, and emerge in interrelationship with the context in which they live.

Structuration theory, developed by Anthony Giddens in the late 1970s and early 1980s, proposes an ontology of the social world that necessitates understanding the concept of occupation as emerging in a particular time and place. It presents a theory of social practices ordered across time and space, which moves beyond either interpretative or structuralist positions, favouring neither the individual nor the social. Rather social systems and individuals are engaged in an ongoing reciprocal relationship of mutual influence. Social systems have structuring properties, rules and resources, which give social practices recognizable forms (Giddens, 1984). Structure is located partly within the individual as habits, pre-reflexive and reflexive motivations, memory traces or knowledgeability (Stones, 2001). Therefore while individuals are not passive actors and are able to be discursively conscious, that is, to reflect on their activities, there are also aspects of the social systems with which they engage that are at a non-discursive level, a level of practical consciousness (Giddens, 1984).

The routinization of practices or actions across time and space (re)produce social systems (Hardcastle, Usher, & Holmes, 2005). The most enduring social systems are institutions and, whether economic, political, or religious, they have a long-term recursive influence on social activity (Giddens, 1984). This is not to support a structuralist understanding of the emergence of everyday life, and the agency of the individual is recognized. However, it is proposed that by examining the nature of the institutions and the practices that they support, it is possible to gain a greater understanding of the nature and characteristics of occupation, as it has developed in its particular context, within a particular world view.

Historico-political perspectives on occupation

Religion

For much of the past 2000 years the Christian church has dominated the regulation of religious practices in the Western world; practices which together with their related beliefs and values, form an integral part of everyday life. Christianity is currently comprised of three major branches: Catholic, Protestant and Eastern Orthodox. In anglophone Western Europe, the dominant religion is Protestantism and in the USA over 45% of the population is Protestant (Kosmin, Mayer, & Keysar, 2001).

Influential in both Protestantism and Catholicism is Augustine's doctrine of original sin.[1] From this doctrine God emerged as anthromorphic, wrathful and punishing. It taught Christians that humanity is irreparably flawed and the guilt of Adam and Eve is inherited by their descendents. The resulting feelings of considerable uncertainty, fear and guilt, have affected attitudes to life and daily activity (Armstrong, 1999).

Protestantism emerged in the sixteenth century as society became restless for new guidance in an era of rising individualism, the emergence of city states in Germany and criticism of old religious practices (Armstrong, 1999). Protestantism placed central emphasis on the conscious, reasoning individual who, through faith guided by the scriptures, would receive justification by grace alone; that is, would be declared by God to be innocent of sin (Gerstner, 1995; Owen, 1823; Tillich, 1937). Such a faith demanded an active individual engaged in an ongoing process of inquiry and reflection (McNeill, 1926). Participation in religious policy-making was also encouraged, while the authority and power of the church was reduced, and fatalism and beliefs in magic were undermined (Delacroix & Nielsen, 2001; Israel, 1966).

Individual responsibility also extended to everyday life as it was thought that the result of true belief was that the former sinner turned to good works (Owen, 1823). Luther further developed this idea through his conception of the *calling*. He taught that

[1] Augustine believed that God had condemned humankind to eternal damnation because of Adam's original sin in the Garden of Eden (Armstrong, 1999).

every person had their place in God's world; each person was called to a particular job or trade, and all of these were of equal value in God's eyes. This led to the idea of working with diligence at a job for which one was suited (Weber, 1958/2003), with intrinsic and heavenly rewards, rather than financial gain (Heffernan, 1989), reflected later in the Protestant work ethic.

As a result of Calvin's teachings, daily activity further developed a tremendously dynamic nature (Maurer, 1924). Calvin extended beliefs in the personal responsibility of every believer but created an unbearable tension between the Calvinists' duty to fulfil God's commandments to the best of their ability and without question, while simultaneously living in fear of Hell and damnation due to the doctrine of predestination. At the same time the church, reduced in power and authority, was unable to offer the comfort of confession or communion (Delacroix & Nielsen, 2001; Israel, 1966). The only possible solution was to consider themselves as one of the chosen and to live accordingly (Maurer, 1924; Weber, 1958/2003). It became necessary for the believer to build an entire way of life based on reason and control (Israel, 1966), where the desires of the individual were subjugated to the will of God.

An ascetic way of life emerged, characterized by intense activity, rationality, hard work and thrift (Delacroix & Nielsen, 2001; McNeill, 1926). Activities that promoted personal pleasure, and heightened sensory and emotional experiences, were severely repressed as they were considered to promote illusions and superstitions, distorting God's world (Weber, 1958/2003). Sexual activity was already disapproved of as the means by which the guilt of Adam was passed on to his descendents (Armstrong, 1999). Recreation, like work and religion, was serious and strenuous with a practical or moral purpose, and involvement in community affairs was encouraged as the community was seen to be one of God's creations. The Puritans insisted on reducing the number of days given over to holidays, demanding that only one day a week be set aside for rest (Schor, 1991).

The Protestant work ethic

From these beliefs and teachings emerged the values and ideals referred to as the Protestant work ethic. Christianity has always promoted a work ethic; the New Testament warns against idleness, drunkenness, orgies and the like: 'they which do such things shall not inherit the kingdom of God' (Galations 5: 21 King James Version). In the sixteenth century, Protestantism took on the work ethic. Luther taught the value of savings, pride in achievement, and that hard work would lead to salvation. Due to belief in the reasoning individual, the idle (unemployed) were seen as deliberate sinners, avoiding following the path to salvation (Bernstein, 1988; Heller, 1991).

Luther's doctrine was reinforced by the economic climate of the sixteenth century in Europe. A 25% increase in population, a rapid increase in inflation, and high unemployment led to huge numbers of beggars in the cities of Europe and particularly Germany. At the same time, increasing numbers of the population moved off the land to work in the rapidly developing factories; work that was frequently boring, dangerous and exhausting. This ethic provided a mechanism to ensure a high level of productivity and a perceived worth in these activities (Heller, 1991). It was also used by employers to enforce long working hours; they warned that idleness bred mischief and radicalism (Schor, 1991).

The Protestant work ethic reinforces respect for, admiration of, and willingness to take part in hard work. It promotes independence, integrity, motivation, loyalty and dependability. It also encourages a person to take responsibility for his or her own actions, to value self-control and ambition but to devalue 'broadmindedness, imagination, equality, pleasure, and a comfortable and exciting life' (Furnham, 1982, p. 277). The Protestant work ethic therefore does more than promote hard work; it promotes attitudes where hard work is valued in and for itself and that one should be the best at what one does (Niles, 1993). Max Weber's (1958/2003) thesis is a primary source of work on the relationship between this ethic and the rise of industrialization, and while this has been criticized (Delacroix & Nielsen, 2001), work continued to be perceived as central to daily life throughout the Western world. It has been suggested that the Protestant work ethic 'has become what Weber described as the most compelling "ethos" in American culture and, arguably, in all human life' (McCourtney & Engels, 2003, p. 134).

Economic structures: Imperialism, capitalism and industrialization

From the sixteenth century, the cities of Europe began to expand rapidly with the wealth and raw materials brought from the new trade routes and later the colonies. The explorers, traders and settlers moving to the colonies and to the 'New World' were men (at least initially) demonstrating independence, initiative and considerable determination.

With the development of technological knowledge, the spatial and temporal face of the Western world changed. With the growth of the industrial city, workers moved off the land to find work in the factories, working under the conditions and according to the demands of production. The majority of workers no longer had any choice over what they would produce or when, selling their labour rather than the results of that labour (Kamenka, 1983). At the same time railways and canals were built, enabling natural resources to be exploited wherever they were found, and linking nations internally and with each other. The industrial revolution was unique in the fundamental changes that it brought to society and people's activities within it (Kamenka, 1983).

Work became strictly ordered, taking place in a specific space and time. The widespread use of fossil fuels made it possible for people to work well beyond the natural boundaries of the day and seasons (Carrasco & Mayordomo, 2005). The traditional intermittent and irregular patterns of labour according to the seasons and the light of the day were no longer necessary (Schor, 1991), and the interweaving of productive, community and family life characteristic of non-industrial societies was lost (Lefebrve, 2008).

The dominant and regulated nature of work imposed an equal structure on non-work occupations. Throughout the nineteenth century workers demanded a shorter working day which led to the '3 × 8' doctrine of the International Labour Movement, a demand for a standardized and uniform time for non-work. By the early twentieth century, an equal division of the day with eight hours each for sleep, work and leisure came to be regarded as a natural and proper order of things (Beckers & Mommaas, 1996). The eight-hour working day was approved in 1919 (General Conference of the International Labour Organization, 1919), cementing the temporal regulation of work and leisure time. This also led to the establishment of regular routines to coordinate the daily activities of the family.

The dominance of work was reinforced by the changing nature of time. With the widespread use of clocks, calendars, schedules and deadlines (Larson & Zemke, 2003), time was no longer a space (Yalmambirra, 2000), but acquired a homogenous nature. Time came to be viewed in economic terms. It could be measured according to the amount of money that it could be transformed into and time that was not marketable was regarded as lost or wasted time (Carrasco & Mayordomo, 2005). A demand for shorter working hours was seen to be 'un-American, indecent, un-profitable, and a threat to prosperity' (Schor, 1991, p. 73).

This dominance of work affected other activities such as household work and child care, many of which have become 'invisible', in economic terms at least (Carrasco & Mayordomo 2005), or with a decreased 'value' in comparison to paid work. This particularly affected women and elderly people, labelling them as the least productive and most dependent members of society (Fast, Dosman, & Moran, 2006).

Leisure, already influenced by Protestant beliefs, was further shaped in response to the dominant and structured nature of work. The social and health problems related to the living conditions in industrial cities led factory owners and other authorities to be concerned to provide appropriate leisure activities to support a fit and healthy workforce. By 1900 in the USA, there had been major public investment in land for parks, sports facilities and swimming pools (Chubb & Chubb, 1981). During the 1920s, a number of international movements promoted adult education, workers' sport and workers' gardens and allotments. The International Labour Organization proposed in 1930 the establishment of an international committee to promote amongst workers 'a wholesome and judicious utilization of their spare time' (Beckers & Mommaas, 1996, p. 212). Employers, such as Henry Ford, saw the provision of leisure activities for the workers as a means of creating new reasons to work, promoting loyalty to the company and to industrial progress (Beckers & Mommaas, 1996), an approach maintained in major American companies for most of the century.

At the same time consumerism emerged with an ever-growing focus on buying leisure products and experiences. This trend worked to reinforce the importance of work and thereby, available income (Schor, 1991), but also to reinforce the concern of authorities for the way the workforce used its leisure time. In the 1950s and 1960s the anticipated decline in working hours and the resulting increase in leisure time was greeted with concern by many. Psychiatrists reported Sunday and Christmas neuroses and Vacation Syndromes and the 'significant danger' leisure posed to many (Csikszentmihalyi & Kubey, 1990), and the American Council of Churches met to discuss spare time (Schor, 1991).

By the 1970s, however, it was clear that work hours would not be reduced. Rather, even longer working hours were the norm. Also evident was a change in attitude to work with the rise of 'post-materialist' values, with a desire for personal fulfilment, self-expression and meaning. Young people started to demand satisfying work (Schor, 1991). Despite this, at the end of the twentieth century Americans continued to work harder and longer hours than ever before. Work continued to be predominant and, as opportunities increased, people continued to want even more in terms of activities, goals and achievements. 'We have become walking resumés. If you're not doing something, you're not creating and defining who you are' (Schor, 1991, p. 23).

Education

Education, both within and outside formal educational institutions, has also been influential in the emergence of Western beliefs, values, norms and habits regarding occupation. Understandings of what is important for a child to learn and what is the best method of teaching, based around knowledge of human development and guided by the contemporary religious, economic and political vision of the citizen, lead to the particular forms of education in any society.

Education was fundamental to Protestantism, which placed particular importance on the individual responsibility of the believer, based on his or her knowledge and understanding of the word of God as delivered in the Bible. This required not only literacy but also thought and reflection. From the seventeenth century, the Puritan settlers of north-eastern America developed schools. For example, the Massachusetts Law (1647), also known as the Old Deluder Satan Act, established compulsory schools in that state. General education was offered to all children until the age of 15, when they entered their calling by becoming an apprentice (de Tocqueville, 1835/1998).

Education was believed to take place not only in the school, but also in the home, shop, neighbourhood and church (Holdzkom, 2006). The ideas of John Locke were influential in a wider understanding of education as being the development of the whole character, ethical values and the work ethic. In a series of essays, Locke discussed his ideas that the mind is a blank slate at birth (*tabula rasa*), and that knowledge is derived through experience and through the good example of others (Pfeffer, 2001; Sass, 2010).

Leading up to, and following the War of Independence and the establishment of the United States, ideas flourished around the importance of the individual citizen to the functioning of the new democracy. Throughout the nineteenth century, there was a rapid expansion of educational establishments, particularly in the northern states. Education was seen to be an important part of nation-building, orientated towards the education of free individuals with Puritan values, able to build a strong, competitive capitalistic economy (Meyer *et al.*, 1979).

Following World War I and concern for the moral character of the youth, conservative Protestantism led the demand for the implementation of character education or moral training in schools. This led to the development of curricular and extra-curricular clubs and activities with the aim of instilling in pupils the traits of 'good American citizens' (Setran, 2005, p. 118). Schools, in a similar way to the factory owners at the same time, came to promote clubs, societies and activities as a way to promote a moral and upstanding way of life, demonstrating again the belief that occupation is influential in character development.

Political structures

From the arrival of the first immigrants in America early in the 1600s, democracy was paramount. The first settlers in the north were Puritans, who moved to America to follow their great dream; to live according to their own opinions and to worship their God in freedom. Participation in civil society, education and opportunities for economic gain were equally available to all. As a result, the prosperity of the state was seen to be a result of their own exertions and public fortune as their own fortune. Americans were active citizens, energetically working in business or industry or buying land in order to improve their fortunes, while morally guided by the Protestant religion (de Tocqueville, 1835/1998). Following independence, an expectation and a demand for active citizens in the new democracy emerged. The Declaration of Independence (1776), and the United States Constitution (1787), are based around and support equality and the rights of all to life, liberty and happiness.

Democracy, together with Protestantism, was also important for the promotion of active involvement in community life. These institutions, due to their structures, offered people an egalitarian and participatory experience, but at the same time encouraged them to join together as free individuals to voluntarily fulfil various social functions, including the care of the poor and needy, and the preservation of public morality (Curtis, Baer, & Grabb, 2001).

In recent years, the emergence of neo-Liberalism has reinforced the importance of individual responsibility and the dominance of independence and productivity (Dossa, 2009). Central importance is given to the free market, while welfare provisions and unions have been dismantled (Mudge, 2008). In the workplace, individuals are expected to be highly competent, flexible and with a range of generic skills that will reduce their reliance on one career or employer (Bourdieu, 1998; Hall & Soskice, 2001). They are encouraged to work harder and under high-stress conditions within a structure of individual performance targets, evaluations and related pay rewards. At the same time, the collective and their support from their team or union, for example, are undermined while there is job insecurity and a real threat of unemployment for all levels of employee (Bourdieu, 1998).

Religious, economic, educational and political institutions have been discussed individually; however, it is obvious that their development and their influences are interlinked and overlapping. Intellectual and scientific movements that have addressed the nature of human beings and their activity have also influenced these institutions. For example, the influence of Humanism and later the intellectual movement known as the Enlightenment supported the idea of the responsibility of the individual for his or her own actions and progress (Wilcock, 2003). Since Descartes the Western self has been seen to be bounded, relatively autonomous and independent and with the ability to pursue its own goals (Sökefeld, 1999). More recently, in the mid twentieth century, the existential philosophers developed ideas around the individual and his or her quest for creating meaning in life that could only be uncovered through action, or being in the world (Daigle, 2004; Pervin, 1960).

From this discussion, it is evident that in Western society activity itself came to have a central place. It was extremely important to be active, and this need to be active came to be particularly directed towards those activities given a higher status, that is, work and serious leisure. The rational individual was self-determining; what one did, and how one did it came to be indivisible from one's faith, morality and character. The purpose of one's activity came under external control and was open to public scrutiny. In addition, the hegemony of industrial time, the privatization of public space and the rise of consumerism led to the 'packaging' of activities into named and distinct time segments that could be bought and sold, changing the more fluid and flexible nature of everyday life of pre-industrial times.

Explicating the historico-political influences on occupation: Examples from Greece

Occupational science was established when the increasing affluence of Western society was enabling people to access a greater number of consumer opportunities than ever before and daily life was becoming increasingly complex (Yerxa, 2000). At the same time, existential philosophies were becoming influential and there was a rise in post-materialistic values leading to a concern for the meaning of life. What people could do, how they do it, and why they do it was of contemporary interest. It is now possible to consider the degree to which the prevailing socio-political discourses around daily activity are evident in conceptualizations of occupation within occupational science. The discussion will particularly focus on understandings of occupation as a particular type of activity, its purpose and temporal characteristics, and its place in the expression and construction of identity, and of the meaning of life. Some examples from Greece will be used to illustrate alternative points of view.[2]

Although contemporary definitions of occupation proposed by occupational scientists are broad, for example, 'all the things that people need, want, or have to do' (Wilcock, 2006, p. xiv), it is also evident that occupations are usually considered to be a particular kind of doing or activity. For example, Yerxa (1993) discussed how occupations are essential to the quality of life experienced. Underpinning this statement is the idea that a certain kind of activity and a certain way of doing it is better than another, and it is this kind of activity that is usually considered to be occupation.

Occupational science takes a view of human beings that places them as central actors in their lives; through self-directed, self-organized, self-initiated occupations (Yerxa, 1993, 2000), to take control (Yerxa *et al.*, 1990), control over their environment (Gray, 1997). Yerxa (2000) commented '*Homo occupacio*, the occupational human, is seized by his or her occupations and in so doing takes possession of his or her world' (p. 91). This view of the active nature of occupation moves beyond a description of the physiological processes required for activity. Rather it reflects the tremendously active, dynamic process of daily life of the good Protestant, which has been reinforced in the twentieth-century character education of the American citizen, together with the individualism characteristic of much of Western society.

In contrast to the USA, Greece has been described as a society with collectivistic features, particularly in its more rural regions (Hofstede & Hofstede, 2005; Triandis, 1989). Gaining independence in 1821 after 400 years of Ottoman rule, it has not undergone a major process of industrialization and the vast majority of the population are Eastern Orthodox Christians. The Orthodox Church is a mystical religion, encouraging reflection and silence within which one can experience the presence of God (Armstrong, 1999). The Orthodox Church did not follow the doctrine of original sin and therefore believers were not burdened with that guilt. All sins can be forgiven and forgiveness is available through the sacrament of confession (Chliaoutakis *et al.*, 2002). There are teachings about certain aspects of daily activity such as caring

[2] Discussion and examples from Greece are based on an ongoing ethnographic study in a small Greek town exploring the daily life and occupations of the inhabitants.

for one's physical health, due to the inter-connectedness of body and soul, and the importance of living as part of the community (Chliaoutakis *et al.*, 2002); however, the tremendous emphasis on activity itself that emerged within the Protestant religion is not evident. Activity is not linked to character formation (although it may be seen as a vehicle for its expression) and educational structures focus particularly on classroom, textbook-based knowledge. Generally, attitudes to activity may be seen to be expressed in the value given to being *metrimenos* (moderate, prudent), to avoiding *agxos* (anxiety) and the belief that too much work and strong emotions are not good for one. Individuals are not compelled to engage in a dynamic self-directed process of taking control, making choices, achieving targets; rather activity takes place in a more contextualized and interrelated way characteristic of more collectivistic societies (Oyserman, Coon, & Kemmelmeier, 2002; Triandis & Gelfand, 1998).

Occupations are said to be purposeful and that purpose has most frequently been categorized as work, leisure and rest or self-care (Christiansen, 1994; Molineux, 2010), while occupations are frequently defined to be chunks or units of activities, classified and named by the culture according to the purpose they serve (Yerxa, 1993). Throughout the occupational literature central importance is given to productivity, work and serious (Stebbins, 2004) leisure occupations.

Primeau (1996) discussed how Protestant values orientated the purpose of daily activity to external, visible and measurable objectives, while the role of industrialization in the emergence of the dichotomy of work and leisure and the dominance given to work has been illustrated. The increasing regulation of occupations into temporal and spatial segments also assisted in identifying, naming and assigning value to specific occupations according to their objective purpose. It has been suggested that occupation may be defined as an individual's specific, non-repeatable doing of an activity (Pierce, 2001).

Occupation, daily activity, is undoubtedly purposeful. However, the purpose of occupation may be enfolded, interwoven, emergent and complex. The purpose may be individual, familial or societal, intrinsic or extrinsic. Occupations in Greece tend to arise as a vehicle for significant aspects of life such as sustaining oneself and one's family (economically and practically), maintaining one's place in one's family group and community, and as a release from daily tensions and stress. Gidden's (1984) description of activity emerging in a continuous flow, spatial and temporal, with multiple influences and unforeseen results, is consistent with the experience of occupation in a Greek town. Social, familial and productive occupations are interwoven temporally and spatially, while the importance or value assigned to them is relative and flexible, dependent on both objective and subjective factors.

Occupation is understood to be linked to the development and expression of identity (Christiansen, 1999; Laliberte Rudman, 2002). Unruh (2004) discussed the concept of occupational identity, which has as its core the individual self with control over its identity and concepts such as self-esteem and personal achievements (Phelan & Kinsella, 2009). This view is consistent with the understanding evident in Western society that morality and character are exhibited in what one does. This is reflected in the question commonly asked on meeting someone 'what do you do?', which is anticipated to give multiple information regarding class, ability and values, that is, an insight into who one is (Unruh, 2004). In Greece it is common, particularly in rural areas, to ask 'whose are you?' referring to kinship lines. Identity, including character, is closely linked to one's family group. In the absence of the Protestant work ethic and Luther's ideas around a calling, work is linked to economic necessity, and while character may be seen to be visible through work and other occupations, they are not perceived to be a vehicle for its formation or expression. Educational institutions, while charged by the constitution to aim for 'moral, intellectual, professional and physical training' and the development of citizens (Hellenic Parliament, 2001), mainly do this through a focus on the transfer of knowledge via the learning of facts, and there are few clubs or organized activities in schools. Entry to higher education is by exam score, and information requested on job application forms is restricted to examination results.

Discussions of the nature of occupation include discussions of temporality. Occupation is described as filling the stream of time (Kielhofner, 2002) and as organizing time (Law *et al.*, 2002). Occupations, when considered as chunks of named activity, imply temporal boundaries, a beginning, a middle and an end (Gray, 1997). These understandings of the temporality of occupation reflect the attitudes that emerged during industrialization; that time is homogenous and that 'time is money'. Time has become an entity, something that should be filled, controlled, organized and importantly, not wasted. As already discussed, temporal, spatial and occupational boundaries in Greece are more flexible and fluid. Many businesses are small and family run, which enables individualized decision-making regarding both timeframes and profit margins. Occupations are not only externally driven but also have a strong subjective component. Fun with one's *parea* (friendship group), relaxation, hanging-out and family-based occupations, are highly regarded and time spent on these is considered time well spent. At the same time, the socially driven or subjective nature of these occupations requires more flexible timeframes in which they may occur.

A core characteristic of occupation is that it carries meaning, in the sense of providing significance to life (Ikiugu, 2005), reflecting the turn against materialism, the questioning of religious beliefs and the influence of existential philosophies in the second part of the twentieth century. It has been argued elsewhere that such understandings of meaning reflect the affluent nature of Western middle-class society (Hammell, 2009). They also reflect the central position given, that is, a consciousness of occupation/activity in Western society. Underpinning much of Greek daily life are core religious beliefs, while over this foundation is a taken-for-granted attitude to what one does, supported by the relatively few choices available to the majority of the population. A good life is primarily related to having good health, for oneself but especially of one's children, to having sufficient income to support yourself and your family, and to a general quality of daily life without major upsets or traumas. Occupation may be a vehicle for these but is not itself the focus.

Conclusion

The concept of occupation as discussed in the occupational science literature had its genesis within the historico-political discourse around activity in the Western world. This is inevitable as occupational scientists, predominantly anglophones, worked to establish and develop the discipline within that world. However, this current conceptualization may limit the potential and expansion of the discipline if occupation continues to be discussed in a way that is not coherent with other world views and with other people's experiences.

However, there are a number of challenges inherent in expanding knowledge and understanding of occupation. It is necessary to leave one's ontological security, to move beyond one's own world view, to open oneself to the experience of other realities. This necessarily entails a process involving insecurity and critique of what one experiences as real. Another challenge is that social reality is expressed through language and the construction of language and reality are interrelated. For example, difficulties in the translation of the word occupation to other languages should be recognized as indicating that occupation does not exist, or is not conceptualized in the same way, in other languages. Another obstacle is the power of anglophone academic discourse. The hegemony of the West due to prestige, ideology and material advantage, has been discussed in relation to occupational therapy (Frank & Zemke, 2008), but also is evident in occupational science. The challenge therefore is to construct a valid dialogue that will enable exploration of occupation in all its complexity and variability throughout the world.

Acknowledgement

This chapter is based upon work undertaken as part of the doctoral studies of the first author at the Faculty of Health & Social Sciences, Leeds Metropolitan University, Leeds, UK. Our sincere thanks to Sally Foster, Director of Studies, for her advice and support.

References

Archer, M. (2000). *Being Human: The Problem of Agency.* Cambridge: Cambridge University Press.

Armstrong, K. (1999). *A History of God.* London: Vintage.

Beckers, T., & Mommaas, H. (1996). The international perspective in leisure research: Cross-national contacts and comparisons. In H. Mommaas, H. van der Poel, P. Bramham & I. Henry (Eds), *Leisure Research in Europe. Methods and Traditions* (pp. 209–43). Wallingford, UK: CAB International.

Berger, P.L., & Luckman, T. (1966). *The Social Construction of Reality.* New York: Anchor Books.

Bernstein, P. (1988). The work ethic: Economics, not religion. *Business Horizons*, **31**, 8–11.

Bourdieu, P. (1977). *Outline of a Theory of Practice* (trans. R. Nice). Cambridge: Cambridge University Press. [Original work published 1972]

Bourdieu, P. (1998). The Essence of Neoliberalism [Electronic version]. *Le Monde.* Retrieved 30 May 2010, from http://www.analitica.com/bitblio/bourdieu/neoliberalism.asp

Carrasco, C., & Mayordomo, M. (2005). Beyond employment. Working time and living time. *Time and Society*, **14**, 231–59.

Chliaoutakis, J.E., Drakou, I., Gnardellis, H. *et al.* (2002). Greek Christian Orthodox ecclesiastical lifestyle: Could it become a pattern of health-related behaviour? *Preventative Medicine*, **34**, 438–5.

Christiansen, C.H. (1994). Classification and study in occupation. A review and discussion of taxonomies. *Journal of Occupational Science: Australia*, **1**, 3–20.

Christiansen, C.H. (1999). Defining lives: Occupation as identity: An essay on competence, coherence, and the creation of meaning. 1999 Eleanor Clarke Slagle lecture. *American Journal of Occupational Therapy*, **53**, 547–57.

Chubb, M., & Chubb, H. (1981). *One Third of Our Time. An Introduction to Recreation Behaviour and Resources*. New York: John Wiley & Sons, Inc.

Cobern, W.W. (1993). *World View, Metaphysics, and Epistemology*. Paper presented at the annual meeting of the National Association for Research in Science Teaching. Retrieved 7 September 2010, from http://www.wmich.edu/slcsp/SLCSP106/SLCSP106.PDF

Csikszentmihalyi, M., & Kubey, R. (1990). *Television and the Quality of Life. How Viewing Shapes Everyday Experience*. Hillsdale, NJ: Lawrence Erlbaum.

Curtis, J.E., Baer, D.E., & Grabb, E.G. (2001). Nations of joiners: Explaining voluntary association membership in democratic societies. *American Sociological Review*, **66**, 783–805.

Daigle, C. (2004). Sartre and Nietzsche. *Sartre Studies International*, **10**, 195–210.

de Tocqueville, A. (1998). *Democracy in America* (trans. H. Reeve). Ware, UK: Wordsworth Editions. [Original work published 1835].

Declaration of Independence. (1776). Retrieved 9 September 2010, from http://archives.gov/exhibits/charters/declaration_transcript.html

Delacroix, J., & Nielsen, F. (2001). The beloved myth: Protestantism and the rise of industrial capitalism in nineteenth-century Europe. *Social Forces*, **80**, 509–53.

Dossa, P. (2009). *Racialized Bodies, Disabling Worlds: Storied Lives of Immigrant Muslim Women*. Toronto: University of Toronto Press.

Fast, J., Dosman, D., & Moran, L. (2006). Productive activity in later life: Stability and change across three decades. *Research on Aging*, **28**, 691–712.

Frank, G., & Zemke, R. (2008). Occupational therapy foundations for political engagement and social transformation. In N. Pollard, D. Sakellariou, & F. Kronenberg (Eds), *A Political Practice of Occupational Therapy* (pp. 111–36). Edinburgh: Churchill Livingstone Elsevier.

Furnham, A. (1982). The Protestant work ethic and attitudes towards unemployment. *Journal of Occupational Psychology*, **55**, 277–85.

General Conference of the International Labour Organization. (1919). *Hours of Work (Industry) Convention*. Retrieved 20 May 2009, from http://www.dsal.gov.mo/law/E1.htm

Gerstner, J. (1995). *Justification by Faith Alone: Affirming the Doctrine by which the Church and the Individual Stands or Falls*. Retrieved 24 May 2009, from http://www.the-highway.com/Justification-Gerstner.html

Giddens, A. (1984). *The Constitution of Society*. Cambridge: Polity Press.

Gray, J.M. (1997). Application of the phenomenological method to the concept of occupation. *Journal of Occupational Science*, **4**, 5–17.

Hall, P.A., & Soskice, D. (2001). An introduction to varieties of capitalism. In P.A. Hall & D. Soskice (Eds), *Varieties of Capitalism* (pp. 1–70). Oxford: Oxford University Press.

Hammell, K.W. (2009). Sacred texts: A sceptical exploration of the assumptions underpinning theories of occupation. *Canadian Journal of Occupational Therapy*, **76**, 6–13.

Hardcastle, M., Usher, K., & Holmes, C. (2005). An overview of structuration theory and its usefulness for nursing research. *Nursing Philosophy*, **6**, 223–34.

Heffernan, N. (1989). *Capital, Class and Technology in Contemporary American Culture*. London: Pluto Press.

Hellenic Parliament. (2001). *Constitution of Greece. As revised by the VIIth Revisionary Parliament*. Retrieved 20 October 2010, from www.nis.gr/npimages/docs/Constitution_EN.pdf

Heller, F. (1991). Reassessing the work ethic: A new look at work and other activities. *European Work and Organizational Psychologist*, **1**, 147–60.

Hofstede, G., & Hofstede, G.J. (2005). *Cultures and Organizations. Software of the Mind*. New York: McGraw-Hill.

Holdzkom, D. (2006). National education policy and popular education: A reconsideration of Cremin's The Genius of American Education. *Journal of Thought*, **41**, 79–83.

Ikiugu, M. (2005). Meaningfulness of occupations as an occupational-life-trajectory attractor. *Journal of Occupational Science*, **12**, 102–9.

Israel, H. (1966). Some religious factors in the emergence of industrial society in England. *American Sociological Review*, **31**, 589–99.

Kamenka, E. (1983). Introduction. In E. Kamenka (Ed.), *Karl Marx* (pp. xi–xlv). Harmondsworth, UK: Penguin Books.

Kielhofner, G. (2002). *Model of Human Occupation: Theory and Practice* (3rd ed.). Philadelphia, PA: Lippincott Williams & Wilkins.

Kosmin, B.A., Mayer, E., & Keysar, A. (2001). *American Religious Identification Survey*. New York: The Graduate Centre of the City University of New York.

Laliberte Rudman, D. (2002). Linking occupation and identity: Lessons learned through qualitative exploration. *Journal of Occupational Science*, **9**, 12–19.

Laliberte Rudman, D., Dennhardt, S., Fok, D. *et al.* (2008). A vision for occupational science: Reflecting on our disciplinary culture. *Journal of Occupational Science*, **15**, 136–46.

Larson, E., & Zemke, R. (2003). Shaping the temporal patterns of our lives: The social coordination of occupation. *Journal of Occupational Science*, **10**, 80–9.

Law, M., Polatajko, H., Baptiste, S., & Townsend, E. (2002). Core concepts of occupational therapy. In E. Townsend (Ed.), *Enabling Occupation: An Occupational Therapy Perspective* (2nd ed., pp. 29–56). Ottawa: Canadian Association of Occupational Therapists.

Lefebrve, H. (2008). *Critique of Everyday Life, Volume I* (trans. J. Moore). London: Verso. [Original work published 1958]

Massachusetts Law of 1647. (1647). Retrieved 20 October 2010, from www.lawlib.state.ma.us/docs/DeluderSatan.pdf

Maurer, H. (1924). Studies in the sociology of religion. I. The sociology of Protestantism. *The American Journal of Sociology*, **30**, 237–86.

McCourtney, A., & Engels, D. (2003). Revisiting the work ethic in America. *The Career Development Quarterly*, **52**, 132–49.
McNeill, J. (1926). The interpretation of Protestantism during the past quarter-century. *The Journal of Religion*, **6**, 504–25.
Meyer, J., Tyack, D., Nagel, J., & Gordon, A. (1979). Public education as nation-building in America: Enrolments and bureaucratization in the American states, 1870–1930. *American Journal of Sociology*, **85**, 591–613.
Molineux, M. (2010). The nature of occupation. In M. Curtin, M. Molineux & J. Supyk (Eds), *Occupational Therapy and Physical Dysfunction: Enabling Occupation* (6th ed., pp. 17–26). Edinburgh: Elsevier.
Mudge, S.L. (2008). The state of the art. What is neo-liberalism? *Socio-Economic Review*, **6**, 703–31.
Niles, F.S. (1993). The work ethic in Australia and Sri Lanka. *The Journal of Social Psychology*, **134**, 55–9.
Owen, J. (1823). *The doctrine of justification by faith through the imputed righteousness of Christ*. Retrieved from http://books.google.com
Oyserman, D., Coon, H.M., & Kemmelmeier, M. (2002). Rethinking individualism and collectivism: Evaluation of theoretical assumptions and meta-analysis. *Psychological Bulletin*, **128**, 3–72.
Pervin, L. (1960). Existentialism, psychology and psychotherapy. *American Psychologist*, **15**, 305–9.
Pfeffer, J.L. (2001). The family in John Locke's political thought. *Polity*, **33**, 593–618.
Phelan, S., & Kinsella, E.A. (2009). Occupational identity: Engaging socio-cultural perspectives. *Journal of Occupational Science*, **16**, 85–91.
Pierce, D. (2001). Untangling occupation and activity. *American Journal of Occupational Therapy*, **55**, 138–46.
Primeau, L. (1996). Work and leisure: Transcending the dichotomy. *American Journal of Occupational Therapy*, **50**, 569–77.
Sass, E. (2010). *American educational history: A hypertext timeline*. Retrieved 6 July 2010, from http://www.cloudnet.com/~edrbsass/educationhistorytimeline.html
Scheurich, J.J., & McKenzie, K.B. (2005). Foucault's methodologies. Archeology and genealogy. In N. Denzin & Y. Lincoln (Eds), *The Sage Handbook of Qualitative Research* (3rd ed., pp. 841–68). Thousand Oaks: Sage.
Schor, J.B. (1991). *The Overworked American: The Unexpected Decline of Leisure*. New York: Basic Books.
Setran, D. (2005). Morality for the "Democracy of God": George Albert Coe and the liberal Protestant critique of American character education, 1917–1940. *Religion and American Culture*, **15**, 107–44.
Sökefeld, M. (1999). Debating self, identity, and culture in anthropology. *Current Anthropology*, **40**, 417–47.
Stebbins, R.A. (2004). *Erasing the line between work and leisure in North America*. Paper presented at the 'Leisure and liberty in North America' Conference. Retrieved 13 July 2010, from http://people.ucalgary.ca/~stebbins/leisurelibertyinnpap.pdf
Stones, R. (2001). Refusing the realism-structuration divide. *European Journal of Social Theory*, **4**, 177–97.
Tillich, P. (1937). Protestantism in the present world situation. *American Journal of Sociology*, **43**, 236–48.

Triandis, H. (1989). The self and social behaviour in differing cultural contexts. *Psychological Review*, **96**, 506–20.

Triandis, H., & Gelfand, M. (1998). Converging measurement of horizontal and vertical individualism and collectivism. *Journal of Personality and Social Psychology*, **74**, 118–28.

United States Constitution. (1787). Retrieved 16 October 2010, from http://www.usconstitution.net/const.html

Unruh, A. (2004). Reflections on: "So... what do you do?" Occupation and the construction of identity. *Canadian Journal of Occupational Therapy*, **21**, 290–5.

Weber, M. (2003). *The Protestant Ethic and the Spirit of Capitalism* (trans. T. Parsons). New York: Dover Publications. [Original work published 1958]

Whiteford, G., Townsend, E., & Hocking, C. (2000). Reflections on a renaissance of occupation. *Canadian Journal of Occupational Therapy*, **67**, 61–9.

Wilcock, A.A. (2001). What is occupational science? *British Journal of Occupational Therapy*, **64**, 412–17.

Wilcock, A.A. (2003). A science of occupation: Ancient or modern? *Journal of Occupational Science*, **10**, 115–19.

Wilcock, A.A. (2006). *An Occupational Perspective of Health* (2nd ed.). Thorofare: Slack.

Yalmambirra. (2000). Black time ... white time: Your time ... my time. *Journal of Occupational Science*, **7**, 133–7.

Yerxa, E. (1993). Occupational science: A new source of power for participants in occupational therapy. *Journal of Occupational Science: Australia*, **1**, 3–9.

Yerxa, E. (2000). Occupational science: A renaissance of service to humankind through knowledge. *Occupational Therapy International*, **7**, 87–98.

Yerxa, E., Clark, F., Frank, G. *et al.* (1990). An introduction to occupational science. A foundation for occupational therapy in the 21st century. *Occupational Therapy in Health Care*, **6**, 1–17.

5

Occupations through the looking glass: Reflecting on occupational scientists' ontological assumptions

Clare Hocking

Looking glasses enable people to see themselves. Aside from fairground mirrors, which deliberately distort the image for comic effect, looking glasses are presumed to provide an accurate reflection. Noting that assumption, Charles Horton Cooley proposed the concept of a 'looking glass self' in 1902 (McIntyre, 2006). That is, in the same way that we check our physical appearance by examining our reflection in a mirror, we learn about other aspects of ourselves by observing people's responses to our appearance and actions, what we say and who we associate with. In simple terms, 'we learn to see ourselves as others see us' (Yeung & Martin, 2003, p. 843), and modify our self-concept to align with the opinions of others. Most influential are the opinions of people we look up to or perceive as having higher status than ourselves. Sociologists and social psychologists propose that even young children have a looking glass self, with some suggesting that people continue to modify their self-concept on the basis of their interactions with others over their lifetime (Yeung & Martin, 2003).

In this chapter, I critically reflect on what occupational scientists and therapists see reflected back to them when they read and refer to published occupational science

Occupational Science: Society, Inclusion, Participation, First Edition.
Edited by Gail Whiteford and Clare Hocking.

research. My intent in undertaking this review of the literature is to seriously consider the possibility that there are attendant limitations in the way occupational scientists have considered and described occupation which have led to distortions in knowledge production. The assumption behind my interrogation parallels Cooley's proposal that individuals readily respond to images of themselves, accepting and integrating the viewpoint of others as real or at least plausible. By extension, current understandings of human occupation based on uni-dimensional representations might be accepted as universal explanations of the norms, forms and value of occupational participation.

Clearly, such non-critical acceptance of a homogenized science of occupation is problematic. The reality is that, to date, occupational science has been subject to a number of biases brought about by its historical circumstances – the relatively small numbers of occupational scientists who are, on the whole, female, middle class, located in Western academic contexts and with a background in occupational therapy practice. For this reason, it is timely that occupation is investigated and understood from multiple ontological standpoints including, for example, as gendered, socio-cultural and socio-economic constructions. The necessity of such a development to the future viability and relevance of occupational science has been noted increasingly in the literature (Dickie, Cutchin, & Humphry, 2006; Molineux and Whiteford, 2011 Pierce *et al.*, 2010). In the following sections, what might be considered within such constructions and what the contribution to the growing corpus of knowledge in occupational science might be is explored.

Gender bias

Attending an occupational science conference immediately confirms that the majority of occupational scientists are female. Less evident is that the majority of participants in occupational science research are also female. Glover's (2009) systematic review of occupational science literature, for example, examined the age distribution and disability status of research participants, but not their gender. Pierce *et al.* (2010), however, noted that 'adult, white women without disabilities' (p. 209) were the most studied group amongst presenters at conferences convened by the Society for the Study of Occupation: USA. Research articles published in the *Journal of Occupational Science* between 2008 and 2010 similarly provide evidence of a bias towards female participants. In the 41 studies where individual self-report was the primary data source, 34 identify the participants' gender. Of those, 12 set out to recruit only women and a further 10 had more female than male participants – sometimes substantially more. Only two studies had exclusively male participants; one reported the retirement experience of Australian farmers, the other participation in skateboarding. Expressed as percentages, 65% of the 34 studies were female dominated, compared to only 24% that were male dominated.

It is easy to claim that the addition of male perspectives is imperative, given previous claims that the purpose of occupational science is to 'explore the construct of occupation in its entirety' (Molke, Laliberte Rudman, & Polatajko, 2004, p. 276) and to capture 'occupation's richness of meaning' (Primeau, 2000, p. 20). However, identifying what might be added, or what is currently missing, is somewhat more complex. For instance, recognizing the underrepresentation of men's occupations, Pierce and her colleagues (2010) advocated 'research exploring male perspectives' particularly among 'sexual minorities, ethnic minorities, and poor working class men' (p. 209). At first sight this suggestion seems wise, in pointing to research participants whose experience of occupation is likely to provide high contrast to current understandings of occupation. Moreover, research along those lines might uncover social inequalities and occupational injustices, which are an increasingly recognized focus for occupational scientists (Whiteford, 2000).

Framing occupational science's favouring of female research participants as a gender equity issue, however, brings a broader perspective. A quick search of the web readily locates definitions of gender bias, such as 'a preference or prejudice toward one gender over the other' (Ellis, 2003) that can be conscious or unconscious, overt or subtle. Its importance is in its consequences; inequalities in resourcing boys and girls sports (Ellis, 2003), the erosion of female literacy rates and increasing poverty (Jacobson, 2005). While discussions of gender bias usually point to discrimination against women, citing failure to consider women's viewpoint or consider the impact any initiative might have on women and children, discrimination against men can be assumed to risk similar outcomes. So, what are the consequences for occupational science of its relative neglect of men's perspectives and experiences of participation in occupation?

To answer that question, I looked to the broader literature. Not surprisingly, it was easy to locate evidence of differences between male and female perspectives of everyday occupations and that those differences make a difference in relation to health and well-being. Klomsten, Marsh and Skaalvik (2005), for example, identified that secondary school students have gendered values that influence their choice of sports activities. Where boys emphasize strength, endurance and competence, girls place higher value on having an attractive face and being slender and flexible. That difference is important to acknowledge because there is accumulating evidence that girls and women have lower participation rates in sport and other physical activities. Encouraging participation might depend on understanding how such stereotyped values arise, or breaking down the perception that 'boys are not able to do graceful and coordinated activities, and girls cannot be tough, hard, and be able to handle pain' (Klomsten *et al.*, 2005, p. 634). Neither of those suggestions – tracing how societal values are imparted to the next generation or understanding the relationship between people's perception of themselves and what they might do – makes sense without the knowledge that different values and perceptions co-exist.

Similarly, Peterson (2004) found that men and women place importance on different aspects of their working lives, with men prioritizing pay, power and authority, while women prioritize relationships, recognition and respect, communication, collaboration and fairness. What's more, men are generally unaware of what is important to women and women overestimate the importance of money, benefits and status to men. There are also differences in the way men and women define and experience a healthy workplace, with men's health status aligned to management practices and supervision and women's health status more influenced by environmental and cultural aspects. Knowledge of these different orientations would usefully inform occupational scientists' research into employment and other productive occupations yet, while some researchers have accessed such literature to make sense of their findings (see, for example, Håkansson & Ahlborg, 2010), others have relied more on reports of women's work experiences (see, for example, Crooks, Stone, & Owen, 2009) or entirely overlooked gender-based differences (see Jakobsen, 2009). The risk in not being informed about gender differences is that researchers may fail to recognize and report the experience of participants of the opposite gender, or misattribute findings. For example, Jakobsen's (2009) finding that women with rheumatism are concerned about being a burden to their co-workers might readily have been interpreted in light of women's valuing of collaboration and fairness. Equally, her participants' emphasis on their supervisors being understanding and supportive is indeed an important aspect of 'the culture of the work environment' (p. 123), but not unique to women with a disability. Recognizing the alignment between the work experiences of women with a disabling health condition and women in general suggests that the experience of men with a disability might be very different – but the nature of those differences has not been investigated.

In terms of gender equity, therefore, occupational science has, arguably, reported a largely feminized account of occupation to date. Such an observation, however, does not apply so much to the research sites occupational scientists choose, in terms of studies undertaken in the private (feminine) sphere rather than the public (masculine) sphere of human activities. There are more recent studies set in workplaces, a refugee camp, or leisure pursuits outside the home than there are of family routines, home-based leisure pursuits and adjustment to disability. Rather, feminine perspectives surface in the analysis of findings. Thus a tiny minority of articles have described masculine perspectives; control, planning and connection with the land and agricultural work (Wiseman & Whiteford, 2009), challenge, skill acquisition, freedom, fear and risk appraisal (Haines, Smith & Baxter, 2010). More typically, occupation is discussed in terms familiar to women. This is perhaps most evident in research with only female participants, where the meaning of occupation is described using terms that align with feminine attributes of being nurturing and gentle. Accordingly, the analysis yields concepts such as occupation as a vehicle for self-expression; participating in an occupation that is respected within one's culture; caring, making a contribution to others, providing a foundation for children, or benefiting society; as maintaining social networks and connection with others; having obligations, meeting others' expectations and concern about being a burden; and learning one's limits and needing empathy (Boerema, Russell, & Aguilar, 2010; Hunter, 2008; Jakobsen, 2009; Shank & Cutchin, 2010).

Taking Pierce *et al.*'s (2010) observation that occupational scientists most often call on people like themselves to participate in their research – able-bodied, adult, white women – my critique can readily be extended to note the relative absence of other groups. Childhood and adolescent perspectives on occupation are infrequent. While refugee and immigrant perspectives are beginning to appear (see, for example, Boerema *et al.*, 2010; Huot & Laliberte Rudman, 2010; Steindl, Winding, & Runge, 2008), the occupations of people from other ethnic and cultural backgrounds, indigenous perspectives and other minority groups have received little attention. Clearly, those perspectives are needed if occupational scientists are to achieve understanding of occupation in its entirety.

The presumption of individualism

Occupational science has both been critiqued as too individualistic in its conceptualization of occupation (Dickie *et al.*, 2006; Hocking, 2000) and defended as appropriately individualistic for a science instigated to support occupational therapy practice (Pierce *et al.*, 2010). To find a path between these divergent claims, I needed to return to the concept of individualism and to consider the impacts of a largely individualistic epistemology.

Individualism itself can be defined as a doctrine or belief about the importance and worth of each person. Looking into the matter more deeply, individualism encompasses three distinct clusters of ideas about equality of rights, economic liberalism and 'the aristocratic cult of individuality, or Romantic individualism' (Swart, 1962, p. 77). Traces of these ideas can be identified in current definitions. The notion of equal rights appears to underpin definitions of individualism that emphasize a belief in the power of individual reason and 'the doctrine of free enquiry' (Encyclopaedia Britannica, 2011), as well as the emphasis placed on individual choice, needs and goals, and assumptions about individuals' right to happiness and privacy. In the United States in particular, this aspect of individualism is expressed in terms of valuing personal freedom and protected by being self-assertive.

Economic liberalism refers to freedom from governmental control, individual ownership of goods and property, and an expectation that individuals will look after themselves. Those ideas align with other definitions of individualism as concerned with 'individual initiative, action and interests' (Merriman-Webster, n.d.), self-reliance, and economic and political independence. Affiliated concepts include the notion of self-help and the American belief that every citizen can rise above his or her circumstances – the vision of the self-made man. Romantic individualism is underpinned by notions of individual genius and self-realization, and the premise that each person develops his or her own personality or character (TheFreeDictionary.com, n.d.). This aspect of individualism is about taking action to assert one's individuality or express one's personality. In Europe it has connotations of individual uniqueness.

Because it highlights the pursuit of individual interests and achievements rather than shared goals, individualism is often contrasted with collectivism, in the sense that collectivist societies emphasize interdependence over independence and individual rights give way to the good of the group (Wikipedia, 2011). From this perspective, individualism is characterized as standing apart, not feeling like an integral part of society, and being primarily motivated by self-interest (Swart, 1962). Early critics of Romanticism and individualism argued that both 'evaded the pressing social issues' (Swart, 1962, p. 83) in selfishly emphasizing individuality and personal development.

Such a critique signals why individualism as a dominant epistemic frame is problematic for occupational science. If the focus is on individuals, their uniqueness, experience and development, occupational scientists will very probably fail to interrogate the complex causations that underpin occupational phenomena; that is, interactions between socio-cultural and religious mores, economics, history and politics and the impacts these have on either supporting, precluding or depriving people of opportunities for occupational participation. It also makes the adoption of a critical lens (Whiteford & Townsend, 2011) through which occupational scientists might consider ideological and structural issues, and the influence these have on power relations in society, more difficult. Accordingly, issues such as occupational deprivation will be explored only in relation to what happens to people who experience it, rather than the forces beyond the individual that bring it about. Human potential will be viewed as self-determined, without acknowledgement of the realities and perceptions that open up or close down possibilities. Insights into ways that social and physical environments might be structured to elicit healthful occupations will not be sought. Rather, participation in healthful occupations will remain a matter of individual choice, personal responsibility and cost.

Having recognized that deliberately or inadvertently ascribing to an individualistic perspective has limitations, the question of whether occupational science is too individualistic remains. Turning back to the recent literature, examples of research with an individualistic focus can be readily identified. For example, a study of the occupations of tertiary students was reported in 2006 (Alsaker *et al.*,2006). While it investigated the occupational patterns of 22 students, the study was individualistic in scope. Each participant was asked about his or her time use in order to discern what is typical of individuals living the life of a tertiary student; their spheres of activity, how much time was dedicated to different kinds of activities, who they spent time with. Conclusions were drawn about the identity-related goals that motivated students' pattern of time use. That is, the inquiry concerns the choices, goals, actions and interests of individual students, and drew conclusions about the 'repertoire of everyday occupations' (Alsaker *et al.*, 2006) that characterize student life in Europe at present. The discourses that influence students' leisure choices (TV watching, exercising) are absent from the discussion. Equally, the societal implications of these future health professionals spending more time, on average, engaged in leisure than education-related occupations are not addressed; neither is the finding that they engage in a narrow and repetitive range of occupations with people of a similar age, yet will be expected to form effective working relationships with people of all ages and diverse backgrounds.

Similarly, other individualistic studies reported in the occupational science literature fail to problematize the topic they address or their findings. Thus an investigation of the meaning of computer use to older adults (Aguilar, Boerema, & Harrison, 2010) recognized the possibility of using electronic technology to stay in touch with family without questioning the social and economic factors that work against visiting. A compelling account of the occupational consequences of weight loss surgery (Wilson, 2010) did not address occupations implied in becoming obese – cultural messages around food provisioning and preparation, or the dining experience. It seems clear that occupational scientists need to move beyond (often romanticized) accounts of individualized experiences if the discipline is to make any contribution to understanding and responding to the occupational issues of people who experience systematic disadvantages and marginalization.

A middle-class world view

In addition to being biased towards female perspectives, research undertaken by occupational scientists has been critiqued as safely 'middle class' (Hammell, 2011). That is, our vision of what is worthy of study is shaped by our own understandings of how people live their lives and what is important. Those understandings are (largely) middle class, because we have not experienced occupation in the context of chronic poverty, systemic unemployment, food insecurity, a dangerous neighbourhood, and so on. To argue this point, let me describe what I mean in using the descriptor *middle class*.

An exact definition is difficult because commentators bring different perceptions of the nature of being middle class – political, economic status, job status, educational attainment or self-perception. Nonetheless, middle-class people can be described as a socio-economic grouping with a 'comfortable' standard of living relative to others in their society and some level of job security. They are characterized by having a conventional lifestyle and beliefs (Random House, 2010). Western sources evidence some consistency in what those beliefs are, and their alignment with bourgeoisie values. Two authoritative sources, the *Oxford Dictionary of Politics* (McLean & Mc Millan, 2003) and Houghton Mifflin's *The New Dictionary of Cultural Literacy* (Hirsch, Kett, & Trefil, 2002) identify a set of values associated with being a responsible citizen, such as respect for private property and the law, and desire for social respectability. Middle-class people are described as having a conservative outlook; holding fast to the sanctity of the family and moral uprightness, and valuing thrift, hard work, material wealth and education. More populist sources add prudence and moderation, neatness and order, ambition, and continual self-improvement (Brooks, 2010).

So, what does it mean to claim that occupational science has a middle-class world view, and why does that matter? Perhaps the first hint of intent to stay within a tidy middle-class set of assumptions about human affairs is present in the earliest definitions of the science. Occupation, the authors claimed, 'enables humans to be economically self-sufficient' and 'daily pursuits are self initiated, goal directed (purposeful), and socially sanctioned' (Yerxa *et al.*, 1989, p. 5). These are the concerns of the middle class; that people are engaged in productive occupations that generate the material resources they need through the organized application of their skills. Such people not only chose for themselves but chose to engage in occupations that have socially sanctioned purposes and, presumably, outcomes. From participation that fits these criteria, through their own effort and as an outcome of their personal development, individuals fulfil their roles, make a contribution, discover meaning, 'and achieve a sense of efficacy' (Yerxa *et al.*, 1989, p. 10).

But what of occupations that are overtly antisocial? Spray-painting tags, a stylized form of graffiti, onto walls and public buildings (Russell, 2008) is one of the few occupations that have direct social costs to have been researched by occupational scientists. Russell's discussion provides insights into the individual benefits and social functions of this occupation, yet those insights are drawn from the work of sociologists, psychologists and anthropologists. Absent from the literature, thus far, are perspectives occupational scientists might bring, such as how people enter and exit this occupation. What are the satisfactions, the adaptive skills? What meanings do taggers ascribe to their art and how is their identity developed relative to it?

What of occupations 'that are likely to be perceived as disgusting or degrading' (Ashforth & Kreiner, 1999, p. 413) in a physical, social or moral sense, or menial occupations that middle-class people would not choose to engage in? Perspectives on menial work tasks are exposed in the popular television programme, *Undercover Boss*. In it, a company owner is set to work alongside employees who perform time-pressured, demanding jobs that are lacking in glamour. The nature of the work is invisible to the 'boss' until he or she arrives and is shown to lack the capacity to complete the task to the required standard. The work is also clearly positioned as necessary to the functioning and profitability of the organization. In the programme, the stigma of doing menial work is resolved when the boss discovers the humanity, skilfulness, intelligence and dedication of the organization's workers. That is, the workers' value to the organization is viewed from a middle-class standpoint. These people do care, and are prepared to work hard to get ahead or support their children.

Just as it is not possible to evaluate a person's well-being if their situation is uncertain (Aldrich, 2011), it is not credible to think that occupational scientists will fully understand occupation until researchers venture beyond these familiar viewpoints, to discover how other people experience the things they do. Discoveries await those who explore occupations that are outside their experience. Questions arising from the discipline's quest to understand the meaning of occupation include how people manage the identity implications of doing low status work. What motivates them to do a good job? Do values such as orderliness, routine, being prudent and considered, or self-improvement have any currency? Taking a less romanticized perspective, what is the experience of a life devoid of productive occupation, whether that comes about because of privilege, choice or circumstance? What of people whose occupations are immoderate, rash, spontaneous, fruitless or chaotic? Studying occupations at the extremes might illuminate ways in which middle-class views of occupation are limited and oppressive, excluding people who are disadvantaged by structural inequities.

As well as occupations that fall outside the experience of the middle classes, or defy middle-class values, occupational scientists might usefully commit to studying familiar occupations performed under conditions of uncertainty or duress. For instance, there has been much discussion in the occupational science literature of occupational patterns and time use. One such is Alsaker *et al.*'s (2006) study of tertiary students, discussed earlier. To extend our understanding of the ways in which people's occupations are patterned, researchers might seek out participants whose daily round of occupations is under stress, for example by living long term in overcrowded housing or dangerous neighbourhoods. There is much to learn. To illustrate that point, consider a study of food-consumption patterns of low-income families in Britain (Dobson *et al.*, 1994). It reported strategies that women use to contain the cost of food; buying the same items each week so they will know how much they are spending, avoiding new products because it would be a waste of money if the family did not eat them, not having a stock of food because family members would help themselves, and when money is really tight, buying only what would be eaten that day. These strategies make perfect sense, but they are not ones I am familiar with. The reason is simple: this is not the life I lead.

A way forward

I have argued that, in the main, occupational science is too slanted towards women's realities and concerns, overly focused on individuals' experiences, and sanitized by middle-class values. On that basis, I have urged occupational scientists to develop their work by engaging with more diverse populations in order to broaden our epistemic basis and the ontologies we may seek to represent – in other words, embrace occupation in all its rich, situated, messy complexity. Until occupational scientists embrace that complexity, the knowledge and perspectives they bring to important questions of health and justice will be partial, reflecting the reality of only a tiny proportion of the world's people.

Achieving the goal of generating knowledge that is not individualistic, sexist or classist will require a mind shift, from ideas that sit comfortably with middle-class assumptions about working hard and being responsible for ourselves, to researchers taking an activist stance and assuming some responsibility relative to the communities with whom we might engage. The responsibility is twofold: creating 'spaces where people can express and give meaning to the world around them' (Denzin & Giardina, 2009, p. 41) and 'giving precedence . . . to the voices of the least advantaged groups in society' (Mertens, Holmes, & Harris, cited in Denzin & Giardina, 2009, p. 12). How might that be achieved? One strategy is to design studies that unsettle established 'truths' about disadvantaged groups. For instance, in New Zealand recipients of social welfare benefits are periodically branded as 'dole bludgers', implying that they take from society with no expectation or demand to give back. Occupational scientists might respond with studies seeking to discover and quantify the *contribution* beneficiaries make. Dissemination of the findings would then be undertaken to achieve maximum media exposure, with the goal of provoking change in public and political sentiment. Taking a more critical stance, occupational scientists might seek to uncover the mechanisms that perpetuate injustices. To paraphrase Denzin and Giardina (2009), an occupational scientist might go beyond studies that have documented instances of occupational deprivation to ask: How do victims of occupational injustice come to accept and even collaborate in maintaining aspects of the system?

Another research strategy to more directly challenge widely held views is termed 'bearing witness', a concept discussed by critical anthropologists. The idea is to bring social (and occupational) injustices to people's attention in ways that invoke a response 'to what was seen, heard, learned, felt and done' (Madison, 2009). Horghagen and Josephsson's (2010) account of a theatre production developed and staged by asylum seekers living in an immigration centre in Norway is an example. Bearing witness opens up the possibility that others will respond. As Durland (cited in Madison, 2009) explained 'a person who bears witness to an injustice takes responsibility for that awareness. That person may then choose to do something or stand by, but he (sic) may not turn away in ignorance' (p. 65).

A third strategy is to undertake studies to directly inform political change. For instance, knowing that people with a disability have the lowest employment rates of any group in society, occupational scientists might conduct case studies to identify workplace practices, policies, attitudes and circumstances that support the inclusion of people with diverse capabilities. The findings would provide a basis for the development of inclusive workplaces, including the design of effective accommodations that would potentially benefit all employees. Similarly, occupational scientists might turn their attention to the health costs of city dwellers' daily commute, the long working hours of the working poor (Shah & Marks, 2004), the impact substandard school environments have on children's performance, or temporal, social and psychological aspects of work known to negatively impact health (Commission to Build a Healthier America, 2009). Alternatively, noting that consumption does not ensure happiness and well-being as much as relationships and community involvement do (Shah & Marks, 2004), occupational scientists might investigate the benefits of volunteering to families and communities. The results would be positioned in relation to consumerism, because engaging in volunteer work displaces other leisure time occupations that involve consumption, and generate knowledge useful for promoting volunteering as a health-promoting occupation. The study would be part of a larger effort to shift health funding into supporting occupations that promote individual and community well-being, and in the longer term, undermine political allegiance to economic growth underpinned by escalating levels of consumption.

These few examples of research topics and questions open possibilities for occupational science researchers to engage in a critical scholarship which has potential to at once inform processes of social change whilst also evaluating impacts from the perspective of those whose occupational needs are often poorly met. In this way, the exciting development of the future for occupational science could be one in which we act as partners in, and agents of, knowledge co-production.

References

Aguilar, A., Boerema, C., & Harrison, J. (2010). Meanings attributed by older adults to computer use. *Journal of Occupational Science*, **17**, 27–33.

Aldrich, R.M. (2011). A review and critique of well-being in occupational therapy and occupational science. *Scandinavian Journal of Occupational Therapy*, **18**, 93–100. doi: 10.3109/11038121003615327

Alsaker, S., Jakobsen, J., Magnus, E. *et al.* (2006). *Journal of Occupational Science*, **13**, 17–26.

Ashforth, B.E., & Kreiner, G.E. (1999) "How can you do it?": Dirty work and the challenge of constructing a positive identity. *Academy of Management Review*, **24**, 413–34.

Boerema, C., Russell, M., & Aguilar, A. (2010). Sewing in the lives of immigrant women. *Journal of Occupational Science*, **17**, 78–84.

Brooks, D. (2010, December 13). Ben Franklin's Nation. *The New York Times Opinion Pages.* Retrieved from http://www.nytimes.com/2010/12/14/opinion/14brooks.html?partner=rssnyt&emc=rss (last accessed 13 June 2011).

Commission to Build a Healthier America. (2009). *Beyond Health Care: New Directions to a Healthier America.* Retrieved from http://www.commissiononhealth.org/Report.aspx?Publication=64498 (last accessed 13 June 2011).

Crooks, V.A., Stone, S.D., & Owen, M. (2009). Multiple sclerosis and academic work: Socio-spatial strategies adopted to maintain employment. *Journal of Occupational Science*, **16**, 25–31.

Denzin, N.K., & Giardina, M.D. (Eds). (2009). *Qualitative Inquiry and Social Justice.* Walnut Creek, CA: Left Coast Press.

Dickie, V., Cutchin, M., & Humphry, R. (2006). Occupation as a transactional experience: A critique of individualism in occupational science. *Journal of Occupational Science*, **13**, 83–93.

Dobson, B., Beardsworth, A., Keil, T., & Walker, R. (1994). *Diet, Choice and Poverty: Social, Cultural and Nutritional Aspects of Food Consumption Among Low-income Families*. London: Family Policy Studies Centre.

Ellis, J. (2003). *What is gender bias?* Retrieved from http://www.wisegeek.com/what-is-gender-bias.htm (last accessed 13 June 2011).

Encyclopaedia Britannica. (2011). Individualism. Retrieved from http://www.Britannica.com/EBchecked/topic/286303/individualism (last accessed 13 June 2011).

Glover, J. (2009). The literature of occupational science: A systematic, quantitative examination of peer-reviewed publications from 1996–2006. *Journal of Occupational Science*, **16**, 92–103.

Haines, C., Smith, T.M., & Baxter, M.F. (2010). Participation in the risk-taking occupation of skateboarding. *Journal of Occupational Science*, **17**, 239–45.

Håkansson, C., & Ahlborg, G. (2010). Perceptions of employment, domestic work, and leisure as predictors of health among women and men. *Journal of Occupational Science*, **17**, 150–7.

Hammell, K.W. (2011). Resisting theoretical imperialism in the disciplines of occupational science and occupational therapy. *British Journal of Occupational Therapy*, **74**, 27–33.

Hirsch, E.D., Kett, J.F., & Trefil, J. (Eds). (2002). *The New Dictionary of Cultural Literacy: Science* (3rd ed.). Boston: Houghton Mifflin Company.

Hocking, C. (2000). Occupational science: A stock take of accumulated insights. *Journal of Occupational Science*, **7**, 58–67.

Horghagen, S., & Josephsson, S. (2010). Theatre as liberation, collaboration and relationship for asylum seekers. *Journal of Occupational Science*, **17**, 168–76.

Hunter, E.G. (2008). Legacy: The occupational transmission of self through actions and artifacts. *Journal of Occupational Science*, **15**, 48–54.

Huot, S., & Laliberte Rudman, D. (2010). The performances and places of identity: Conceptualizing intersections of occupation, identity and place in the process of migration. *Journal of Occupational Science*, **17**, 68–77.

Jacobson, J.L. (2005). *Gender Bias: Roadblock to Sustainable Development*. Retrieved from http://feminism.eserver.org/gender/cyberspace/gender-bias-causes-poverty.html (last accessed 13 June 2011).

Jakobsen, K. (2009). The right to work: Experiences of employees with rheumatism. *Journal of Occupational Science*, **16**, 120–7.

Klomsten, A.T., Marsh, H.W., & Skaalvik, E.M. (2005). Adolescents' perceptions of masculine and feminine values in sports and physical education: A study of gender differences. *Sex Roles*, **52**, 625–36.

Madison, D.S. (2009). Dangerous ethnography. In N. K. Denzin & M.D. Giardina (Eds), *Qualitative Inquiry and Social Justice* (pp. 187–97). Walnut Creek, CA: Left Coast Press.

McIntyre, L. (2006). *The Practical Skeptic: Core Concepts in Sociology* (3rd ed.). New York: McGraw Hill.

McLean, I., & McMillan, A. (Eds). (2003). *The Concise Oxford Dictionary of Politics* (3rd ed.). Oxford: Oxford University Press.

Merriam-Webster. (n.d.) Individualism. In *Merriam-Webster's online dictionary*. Retrieved from http://www. merriam-webster.com/dictionary/individualism (last accessed 13 June 2011).

Molineux, M., & Whiteford, G. (2011). Occupational science: Genesis, evolution and future contribution. In E. Duncan (Ed.), *Foundations for Practice in Occupational Therapy* (2nd ed.). London: Elsevier.

Molke, D.K., Laliberte Rudman, D., & Polatajko, H.J. (2004). The promise of occupational science: A developmental assessment of an emerging academic discipline. *Canadian Journal of Occupational Therapy*, **71**, 269–81.

Peterson, M. (2004). What men and women value at work: Implications for workplace health. *Gender Medicine*, **1**, 106–24.

Pierce, D., Atler, K., Baltisberger, J. *et al.* (2010). Occupational science: A data-based American perspective. *Journal of Occupational Science*, **17**, 204–15.

Primeau, L. (2000). Divisions of household work, routines, and child care occupations in families. *Journal of Occupational Science*, 7, 19–28.

Random House. (2010). Middle class. In *Random House Word Menu*. Retrieved from http://www.answers.com/topic/middle-class (last accessed 13 June 2011).

Russell, E. (2008). Writing on the wall: The form, function and meaning of tagging. *Journal of Occupational Science*, **15**, 87–97.

Shah, H., & Marks, N. (2004). *A Well-being Manifesto for a Flourishing Society: The Power of Well-being*. London: New Economics Foundation.

Shank, K.H., & Cutchin, M.P. (2010). Transactional occupations of older women aging-in-place: Negotiating change and meaning. *Journal of Occupational Science*, **17**, 4–13.

Steindl, C., Winding, K., & Runge, U. (2008). Occupation and participation in everyday life: Women's experiences of an Austrian refugee camp. *Journal of Occupational Science*, **15**, 27–35.

Swart, K.W. (1962). Individualism in the mid-nineteenth century (1826–1860). *Journal of the History of Ideas*, **23**, 77–90.

TheFreeDictionary. (n.d.) *Individualism*. Retrieved from http://www.thefreedictionary.com/individualism (last accessed 13 June 2011).

Whiteford, G. (2000). Occupational deprivation: Global challenge in the new millennium. *British Journal of Occupational Therapy*, **63**, 200–4.

Whiteford, G., & Townsend, E. (2011). A participatory occupational justice framework 2010: Enabling occupational participation and inclusion. In F. Kronenberg, N. Pollard & D. Sakellariou (Eds), *Occupational Therapy without Borders: Towards an Ecology of Occupation-based Practices* (2nd ed., pp. 65–84). Marrickville, Australia: Elsevier.

Wikipedia. (2011). *Collectivism*. Retrieved from http://en.wikipedia.org/wiki/Collectivism (last accessed 13 June 2011).

Wilson, L.H. (2010). Occupational consequences of weight loss surgery: A personal reflection. *Journal of Occupational Science*, **76**, 47–54.

Wiseman, L., & Whiteford, G. (2009). Understanding occupational transitions: A study of older rural men's retirement experiences. *Journal of Occupational Science*, **16**, 104–9.

Yerxa, E.J., Clark, F., Jackson, J. *et al.* (1989). An introduction to occupational science. A foundation for occupational therapy in the 21st century. *Occupational Therapy in Health Care*, **6**, 1–17.

Yeung, K-T., & Martin, J.L. (2003). The looking glass self: An empirical test and elaboration. *Social Forces*, **81**, 843–79.

Part III

Ways of knowing occupation

6 Knowledge paradigms in occupational science: Pluralistic perspectives

Elizabeth Anne Kinsella

Critical epistemological discussions are necessary for the thoughtful advancement of the knowledge base in occupational science. Such conversations can shape how knowledge advances and the directions taken in the field. Yet significant discussions about the philosophical foundations of knowledge paradigms, and how disciplinary knowledge proceeds, are at an early stage in the field of occupational science. In this chapter I draw on various philosophies and philosophers of science to contend that occupational scientists' capacity to reflexively consider the knowledge we produce and the paradigms we embrace is an important collective responsibility at this point in our history.

I begin with a consideration of occupational science as an epistemic community. The term *epistemic community* refers to a knowledge-producing community, such as that constituted by occupational scientists, who apply their standards of credibility to knowledge claims. I draw upon Thomas Kuhn's (1962, 1977) view that scientists use epistemic values to weigh theory choice and to make knowledge commitments. Epistemic values inform the judgements about the utility of a theory and include consideration of its accuracy, consistency, scope, simplicity and fruitfulness. Next, the work of Jürgen Habermas is considered to examine three major knowledge paradigms that have been influential in social science, and which he contends are related to human interests. Following this, I (i) consider the philosophical distinctions between technical and interpretive/critical research, (ii) propose that occupational scientists embrace pluralistic knowledge paradigms, and (iii) examine the role of epistemic reflexivity in advancing knowledge in occupational science.

Occupational Science: Society, Inclusion, Participation, First Edition.
Edited by Gail Whiteford and Clare Hocking.

Occupational science as an epistemic community

In thinking about how knowledge is generated and utilized it is useful to consider the work of Thomas Kuhn, an influential philosopher of science, Kuhn (1962), in his historical studies of how science proceeds, has demonstrated that theory choice, and hence disciplinary knowledge production, involves a social process tied to the judgements that members of epistemic communities make. The Kuhnian view is that theories are parts of knowledge paradigms, constantly shifting based on the predominant values that epistemic communities share and bring to decisions about which theories to adopt. Epistemic communities such as those constituted by occupational scientists, apply their standards of credibility, and epistemic values, to theory choice, yet these constantly shift in response to changes in the predominant values in the field. *Epistemic culture* refers to the particular practices that create and warrant knowledge claims within an epistemic community (Knorr-Cetina, 1999); epistemic culture is also a dynamic entity, which shifts as the actual practices within an epistemic community change.

Epistemic values in occupational science

In his widely read contributions to the philosophy of science, Thomas Kuhn has revolutionalized conceptions of how science proceeds. The following discussion draws from Kinsella and Whiteford's (2009) consideration of the importance of Kuhn's work for conceptualizations of how science proceeds in the occupation-based professions. Kuhn's book, the *Structure of Scientific Revolutions,* has become a seminal contribution to the philosophy of science, and to ongoing debates about what counts as knowledge in the sciences. According to Kuhn (1962), science proceeds as members of epistemic communities make judgements about which theories to adopt and which theories to discard. Collections of theories may be viewed as knowledge 'paradigms', and come to represent the dominant ideas valued by the greatest number of scientists in a field. A cumulative theoretical shift amounts to a paradigm shift. The notion of paradigm was popularized by Kuhn and has been taken up in a number of distinct ways. It can refer to the constellation of beliefs, values, techniques and so on that are shared by the members of a given epistemic community (Kuhn, 1996). Paradigm has also come to refer to 'knowledge paradigms', which represent epistemological stances that inform assumptions about the nature of knowledge (Guba & Lincoln, 1994, 2005). Through his historical analysis of how science proceeds, Kuhn highlighted how scientists shift allegiances from one theory to another, and when this involves a collection of theories, the shift is from one paradigm to another. Transfers of allegiance from theory to theory, or from paradigm to paradigm are more like 'conversions' than a matter of solely building on existing stocks of knowledge and viewing them as cumulative. New knowledge paradigms can emerge from a collection of theories completely distinct, irreconcilable and unrelated to an old paradigm or previously dominant way of seeing the world within a particular discipline. An example of an emerging paradigm shift in occupational science in recent years might be reflected in the shift from scholarship that takes the individual as the predominant focus in the study of occupation, to emerging scholarship that focuses to a greater extent on collective, social and systemic issues as central considerations in the study of human occupation (Christiansen & Townsend, 2010; Dickie, Cutchin, & Humphry, 2006; Fogelberg & Frauwirth, 2010; Molineux & Whiteford, 2006).

Kuhn contended that decisions about theory choice are not neutral, rather they are complicated as members of epistemic communities weigh values in making choices about theories. Kuhn (1977) described five characteristic or epistemic values (accuracy, consistency, scope, simplicity, and fruitfulness) that communities of specialists typically weigh in deciding what counts as knowledge and whether or not to embrace a particular theory. From this perspective, occupational scientists may be viewed as constituting an epistemic community whose judgements inform the theories they adopt, the literature that is published, and the ways in which science proceeds in the discipline.

While arguing that accuracy, consistency, scope, simplicity and fruitfulness are standard criteria for evaluating the adequacy of a theory, Kuhn maintained that these criteria are not precise, for two reasons. First, each of the criteria is imprecise in that individuals may differ in their application to concrete cases, thus the judgement of scientists plays a role in deciding what theories are adopted, utilized or rejected within a particular field. Second, when deployed together, these values often conflict with one another. For instance, one criterion such as accuracy may dictate the choice of a particular theory, while another criterion such as scope may dictate the choice of its competitor. Therefore, the judgements of individuals within epistemic communities are an important consideration with respect to how science proceeds. Kuhn (1977) wrote 'When scientists must choose between competing theories, two men [or women] fully committed to the same list of criteria for choice may nevertheless reach different conclusions' (p. 324).

Theory choice, in Kuhn's view, is not a neutral process. As he wrote in *The Structure of Scientific Revolutions*:

> *There is no neutral algorithm for theory-choice, no systemic decision procedure which, when properly applied, must lead each individual in the group to the same decision. In this sense it is the community of specialists rather than its individual members that makes the effective decision.... What one must understand ... is the manner in which a particular set of shared values interacts with the particular experiences shared by a community of specialists to ensure that most members of the group will ultimately find one set of arguments rather than another decisive.* (Kuhn, 1962, p. 200)

Furthermore, Kuhn argued that the epistemic values are not fixed, others may play a role, and they may vary from community to community. Kuhn in effect argued that communication between proponents of different theories is inevitably partial, that what each individual takes to be fact depends, in part, on the epistemic values that he or she espouses.

This discussion raises a number of questions for occupational scientists. What values do occupational scientists hold with respect to what constitutes knowledge? In what ways might they critically consider and make explicit the epistemic values that inform their community, the consistency of these values in light of the theories adopted, and the implications for the disciplinary knowledge that is generated and utilized? If for instance, occupational scientists value the study of everyday occupation and the lived experiences of individuals, societies and communities in context, what approaches to knowledge generation might they adopt to integrate these value commitments and human interests into research practices? If social justice and the critique of oppressive, exploitative, non-inclusive practices are valued, what are the implications for how occupational scientists approach knowledge generation? What are the possibilities? How might occupational scientists make explicit the epistemic values that inform the quest for disciplinary knowledge, and walk the walk of these values in term of how they judge theories and produce knowledge in occupational science? Given growing interest in occupational science, the growth of the discipline as a unique field of study, and emerging conversations concerning appropriate epistemological foundations in the field (Aldrich, 2008; Barber, 2006; Cutchin *et al.*, 2008; Dickie, Cutchin, & Humphry, 2006; Fogelberg & Frauwirth, 2010; Hocking, 2009; Molke, 2009; Rudman *et al.*, 2008), the time is perhaps right for occupational scientists to critically consider the significance of pluralistic knowledge paradigms, and the consequent diversity of criteria for validation of knowledge claims in occupational science.

Knowledge paradigms

In his influential text *Knowledge and Human Interests,* Habermas (1971) argued that all knowledge claims are tied to human interests. Habermas identified three categories of science, which others have referred to as knowledge paradigms (Guba & Lincoln, 1994), which he viewed as tied to specific knowledge-constitutive interests. According to Habermas (1971), the *empirical-analytical sciences* may be seen as incorporating technical cognitive interests; the *historical-hermeneutic sciences* incorporate interests aimed at human understanding reflective of practical interests; and the approach of a *critically oriented science* which incorporates emancipatory-cognitive interests (Habermas, 1971, p. 308).

In the empirical-analytic science the frame of reference against which the meaning of possible statements is judged establishes rules both for the construction of theories and for their testing. Theories are seen to 'comprise hypothetico-deductive connections of propositions, which permit the deduction of lawlike hypothesis with empirical content' (Habermas, 1971, p. 308). From Habermas' perspective the *human interests* that guide this science are *technical.*

In contrast to empirical-analytic science, interpretive science draws on the historical-hermeneutic sciences. In this conception the meaning of the validity of propositions is not constituted in the frame of reference of technical control (Habermas, 1971). Rather, access to the facts is provided by understanding of meaning, rather than by observation. The verification of law-like hypotheses in the empirical-analytic sciences has its counterpart here in the hermeneutic interpretation of texts. Hermeneutic understanding is always mediated through the interpreter's understanding. Habermas (1971) suggested that *human interests* in the hermeneutic tradition are of a *practical* nature.

Finally, a critical social science, according to Habermas (1971), is not satisfied with the goal of producing nomological (law-like, normative) knowledge. Rather a critical social science is concerned with determining when theoretical statements express ideologically frozen relationships that can in principle be transformed. Critical social science directs critique at the possibility of pure objectivism within the sciences. It seeks to unveil the assumptions embedded within knowledge generation processes, and to make explicit the connection between knowledge generation and human interest. Habermas suggested that the *human interests* that guide critical social science are *emancipatory*.

While Habermas is best known for highlighting the philosophical distinctions between these three forms of science and the interests that drive them, the dichotomies that such a conception sets up between technical, interpretive and critical perspectives are sometimes criticized (Alexander, 2006; Bernstein, 2002; Gadamer, 1996; Howe, 1998; Kinsella, 2006). Gadamer, for instance, objected to Habermas' casting of hermeneutics as only concerned with practical interests and defended the universality of the hermeneutical problem and its application to emancipatory interests (Bernstein, 2002; Kinsella, 2006). Bernstein (2002) summarized this argument:

> *[Gadamer] charges Habermas with succumbing to the worse utopian illusions of the Enlightenment in his attempt to delineate an independent domain of the "new" critical social sciences. Gadamer does not reject the idea of emancipation. He even agrees that it is implicit in Reason itself. But it is not an independent cognitive interest. Rather, it is already intrinsic in hermeneutic understanding.* (p. 271)

In addition, a number of scholars have pointed out that if one adopts a Kuhnian perspective to science, then the differences between technically oriented and interpretive approaches to research are less significant than they have been made out to be (Alexander, 2006; Howe, 1998; Mishler, 1990). Both perspectives require transparency about the research process and explication of the situatedness of the researcher with respect to the production of knowledge. In addition, both rely on similar epistemic values, and the judgements of communities of scientists for the advancement of knowledge. Nonetheless, the work of Habermas has been highly influential in supporting the call for recognition and development of increasingly diverse knowledge paradigms in social science (Guba & Lincoln, 1994, 2005). These knowledge paradigms have been widely adopted by various scholars as frameworks to socially oriented research; some of which are summarized in Table 6.1.

Technical, interpretive and critical knowledge paradigms

Historically, the predominant and taken-for-granted knowledge paradigm in Western societies has been the technical or empirico-analytic science paradigm. This paradigm has drawn on primarily positivist or post-positivist assumptions about what constitutes valid knowledge. Over time a number of philosophically grounded epistemological turns such as the interpretive turn (Hiley, Bohman, & Shusterman, 1991; Rabinow & Sullivan, 1987; Taylor, 1987), the linguistic turn (Rorty, 1979), and the dialogic turn (Camic & Joas, 2004), as well as critical philosophy's critiques of technical knowledge paradigms (Foucault, 1972, 1980; Gramsci, 1971; Habermas, 1971; Horkheimer, 1982; Horkheimer & Adorno, 1972; Lyotard, 1979; Marx, 1964), have challenged traditional knowledge paradigms and opened avenues for interpretive and critical social science.

Table 6.1 Knowledge paradigms

	Technical		Interpretive	Critical	
Habermas (1971)	Empirical-Analytic		Historical-Hermeneutic	Critical-Emancipatory	
Crotty (2003)	Objectivism		Constructionism	Subjectivism	
Guba and Lincoln (2004)	Positivism	Post-Positivism	Constructivism	Critical	
Ponterotto (2005)	Positivism	Post-Positivism	Interpretive	Critical	
Kezar (2004)			Hermeneutic/ Interpretive	Critical	Post-modernism

Positivism/post-positivism

During the course of the nineteenth century the idea of the scientific method, adherence to which guaranteed truth, became widespread. Various fields, in an attempt to legitimate and professionalize their status, embraced objective conduct and scientific method as their modus operandi (Natter, Schatzki, & Jones, 1995). From the middle of the nineteenth century and continuing into the twentieth, a cadre of scientists and philosophers attempted to codify an objective scientific method and thereby provide an epistemological blueprint for the human sciences. Among most scholars there was little doubt that the human sciences should adopt such an approach. Use of objective scientific method as an approach to human sciences reached a highpoint in the 1930s in the epistemological treaties of the Vienna school of theorists (e.g., Karl Popper, Rudolf Carnap, and Otto Neurath), whose 'nomological-deductive' method informed epistemological discussions well into the 1970s (Natter *et al.*). As Kezar (2004) pointed out, during the greater part of the twentieth century the technical scientific method has dominated.

> *As the social sciences absorbed the assumptions of the physical/natural sciences in the 1800s, traditional philosophical questioning about the nature of existence and humankind (ontology), how we know and what constitutes knowledge (epistemology), became marginalized. Instead, one set of assumptions – scientific paradigm – dominated the academy.* (Kezar, 2004, p. 42)

In the last century and particularly in the last 40 years, a number of important philosophical critiques have been launched about the positivist assumptions upon which social and scientific theories and foundational knowledge have been based.

Critiques of the technical paradigm

The philosophical critiques that highlight limitations of knowledge claims within positivist knowledge paradigms argue for alternative approaches to knowledge generation and validation. These philosophical perspectives variously underpin a contention by many different thinkers that 'positivist science's age-old claims to certainty and objectivity cannot be sustained and the findings of natural science are themselves social constructions and human interpretations, albeit a particular form of such constructions and interpretations' (Crotty, 2003, p. 71). A number of these philosophical perspectives inform alternative conceptions of knowledge within interpretive and critical science and offer further avenues for occupational scientists to explore, as scholarship in the field advances. Although an extensive review of these philosophical perspectives is beyond the scope of this chapter, it is important to note that challenges to positivist science, and the presentation of alternative conceptions of what constitutes valid knowledge claims are posited within an array of fields. These are summarized below.

Philosophical foundations of interpretive and critical knowledge paradigms include:

- Anti-foundational philosophy (Rorty, 1979; Ryle, 1949; Taylor, 1991),
- Philosophy of science (Feyerabend, 1975, 1993; Kuhn, 1962),
- Constructivist philosophy (Golinski, 1998; Goodman, 1978; Goodman & Elgin, 1988; Gould, 2003; Kukla, 2000),
- Phenomenological philosophy (Hegel, 1977; Heidegger, 1962–1977; Husserl, 1931–1999; Levinas, 2001; Merleau-Ponty, 1962),
- Social phenomenology (Schutz, 1967, 1970),
- Hermeneutic philosophy (Gadamer 1976, 1996; Ricoeur, 1974–1981),
- Philosophical linguistics (Bakhtin, 1981),
- Pragmatic philosophy (Dewey, 1938; Elgin, 1997; Mead, 1934, 1964; Rorty, 1979),
- Action science (Argyris, 1994; Argyris, Putnam, & Smith, 1985; Bourdieu, 1990, 1998; Lewin, 1951, 1997),
- Social theory/philosophy (Bourdieu & Wacquant, 1992; Dilthey, 1976; Freire, 1970, 1989; Ralston Saul, 1992; Toulmin, 1990; Weber, 1949),
- Social constructionist theory (Berger & Luckman, 1967; Burr, 1995; Gergen, 1994, 1999; Hacking, 1999; Parker, 1998; Potter, 1996; Shotter, 1993a, 1993b),
- Sociology of scientific knowledge (Ashmore, 1989; Latour & Woolgar, 1986),
- Critical theory (Adorno, 1973, 1984; Arato & Gebhardt, 1982; Benhabib, 1986; Connerton, 1980; Gramsci, 1971; Habermas, 1971–1984/1987; Horkheimer, 1982; Horkheimer & Adorno, 1972; Hoy & McCarthy, 1994),
- Marxist theory (Marx, 1961–1964; Marx & Engels, 1937),
- Feminist philosophy of science (Alcoff & Potter, 1993; Code, 1991; Collins, 1991; Haraway, 1991; Harding, 1987, 1991; Harding & Hintikka, 1983; Hekman, 1990; Longino, 1990, 2001; Stanley, 1990; Stanley & Wise, 1993),
- Post-structuralist philosophy (Dreyfus & Rabinow, 1982; Foucault, 1972–1980),
- Post-modern philosophy (Derrida, 1976, 1978; Lyotard, 1979), and
- Post-colonial theory (Collins, 1991; Said, 1978; Spivak, 1990).

Philosophical differences between technical and interpretive/critical research

Writing and scholarship that locates itself in interpretive/critical knowledge paradigms has proliferated to such an extent that some might claim there has been a revolution.

Snape and Spencer (2003) contended that such approaches 'were developed to overcome some of the perceived limitations of the prevailing [positivist] methods used to study human behaviour' (p. 5). As highlighted in the list of perspectives presented above, interpretive and critical scholarship may be informed by a number of distinct schools of philosophy. These schools frequently adopt different epistemic criteria with respect to how knowledge claims are judged to be valid.

Interpretive and critical scholarship might be viewed as complementing traditional approaches to knowledge generation. Such scholarship is informed by unique philosophical and theoretical perspectives, which imply distinct assumptions about what constitutes legitimate knowledge. Additionally, interpretive and critical scholarship frequently draws attention to dimensions, such as human practices, which are considered important to knowledge generation. Interpretive and critical approaches often problematize the idea that there is one objective, value free, factual truth that can be found, and work to make transparent the assumptions and practices that underpin how knowledge is constructed. Such approaches distinguish between research that focuses on technical knowledge, understanding, and social change. There are a number of arguments within the philosophy of science that inform the epistemological roots of, and choices about, research paradigms. Interpretive and critical researchers bring to the foreground various dimensions which are implicated in the construction of knowledge. These might include attention to philosophical and epistemic debates concerning how the following dimensions are implicated in the generation of knowledge:

- The inner lifeworld and subjectivities of persons,
- The role of the body as a medium of perception,
- Reflexive attention to processes of interpretation,
- The complexity of context,
- The positionality of scholars,
- The relationship of the researcher to the researched,
- The relationship between objectivity and subjectivity,
- The distinction between fact and value,
- The distinction between explanation and understanding,
- Issues of language and discourse,
- The ethics of representation and voice,
- The complex social dimensions of human life,
- Issues of politics, power, culture and ideology,
- Consideration of gender, race, and sexual orientation, and
- Consideration of knowledge generation as a social practice.

These topics, while not exhaustive, represent substantive philosophical conversations of importance to conceptions of what constitutes legitimate approaches to knowledge generation in occupational science. The values that members of a particular discipline (such as occupational science) adopt, both individually and collectively, will guide their choices about approaches to knowledge generation that are valued in the discipline (Kinsella & Whiteford, 2009; Kuhn, 1962). Currently such conversations are for the most part implicit in occupational science, suggesting that more explicit attention to the philosophical foundations informing individual and collective assumptions about knowledge generation are important locations for future scholarly dialogue in the field.

Given that occupational scientists are largely concerned with studying everyday occupations in context, and that social, political, economic and cultural conditions are of predominant importance in everyday occupation (Christiansen & Townsend, 2010; Fogelberg & Frauwirth, 2010; Hocking, 2009), interpretive and critical approaches offer significant epistemological frameworks for advancing the knowledge base of the field precisely because they draw attention to complexity and context as has been called for in research practices in occupation science (Darnell, 2002; Fogelberg & Frauwirth, 2010; Hocking, 2009; Rudman *et al.*, 2008). Furthermore, such approaches allow for philosophical consistency in research practices, with the values that occupational scientists espouse, and/or for identification of the irreconcilable gaps and tensions (Darnell, 2002) that serve as invitations for epistemic dialogue. Making such conversations explicit has the potential to inform the values and the research practices that occupational scientists adopt.

Epistemological pluralism

Recently in occupational science there have been a number of healthy debates about which philosophical position should inform the discipline. For example scholars have argued the relative merits of: pragmatist (Dickie *et al.*, 2006) versus phenomenological philosophical foundations (Barber, 2006); individual (Barber, 2006) versus socially oriented perspectives (Dickie *et al.*, 2006; Fogelberg & Frauwirth, 2010; Hocking, 2009; Molineux & Whiteford, 2006); transactional (Aldrich, 2008) versus complexity theory (Fogelberg & Frauwirth, 2010); universal versus culturally oriented perspectives (Darnell, 2002); and neutral versus critically oriented frameworks (Molke, 2009) to name a few. While these are important discussions, I suggest that what the emerging discipline of occupational science requires is not a faithful commitment to a single philosophical foundation, but rather the capacity to engage ongoing dialogues within its epistemic community, to deepen the philosophical discourse, and to embrace epistemological pluralism which is inclusive of knowledge claims informed by *different* philosophical traditions. As an example, the debate between whether pragmatism or phenomenology or transactionalism or complexity theory should inform occupational science is perhaps misplaced; each offer a particular philosophical lens through which to engage the study of human occupation, each represents a variant of interpretive or critical research (if one adopts Habermas' framework, presented earlier) that garners useful and distinct knowledge. Likewise, the critique of individualism in occupational science (Dickie *et al.*, 2006), while important from the perspective of promoting inclusion of socially and culturally oriented perspectives in our scholarly discourse, could perhaps be redirected toward the elicitation of generative dimensions of *both* socially oriented and individually oriented philosophical perspectives. Rather than arguing for one perspective *over* the other, a generative avenue might be to explore the relative merits and limitations to knowledge generation that *each one offers* to scholarship in the field.

I suggest that the philosophical grounding of occupational science should not be chosen *carte blanche*, and that any to attempt to colonize its philosophical foundations is both dangerous and limiting in terms of the future growth of the discipline. Rather, I propose that if the discipline is to thrive and mature, occupational scientists need to welcome diverse and pluralistic philosophical positions, and the consequent diversity of theoretical positions, and approaches to knowledge generation that they invoke. In addition, I suggest that increased attention to deep philosophical work in occupational science and the consequent emergent epistemological conversations is essential as a foundation for future scholarship. The philosophical perspectives informing the science in research practice should reflect the philosophical assumptions about knowledge that inform a particular study and the types of questions that drive the inquiry. Philosophical foundations need not be mutually exclusive, or set up in tension or competition with one another; rather they may be seen as offering a multiplicity of distinct frames through which to enrich the study of occupation.

Epistemic reflexivity

Epistemic reflexivity offers a useful way of thinking critically about knowledge generation within a field (Kinsella & Whiteford, 2009), and is relevant to occupational science. The following discussion draws from and elaborates Kinsella and Whiteford's consideration of epistemic reflexivity as a concept of importance for the occupation-based disciplines.

Bourdieu coined the phrase *epistemic reflexivity*, to denote critical reflection upon the social conditions under which disciplinary knowledge comes into being and gains credence (Bourdieu & Wacquant, 1992). For Bourdieu, reflexivity 'extends beyond the experiencing subject to encompass the organizational and cognitive structure of the discipline' (Bourdieu & Wacquant, 1992, p. 40). Bourdieu urged academics to recognize the specific traditions within which they work and the ways in which such social traditions contribute to knowledge construction (Bourdieu & Wacquant, 1992). Sandywell (1996) elaborated, defining reflexivity as the 'act of interrogating interpretive systems' (p. xiv). Epistemic reflexivity carefully interrogates the very conditions under which knowledge claims are accepted and constructed. Reflexivity recognizes the sociality of the process of knowledge generation and the role of members of epistemic communities in the process. For reflexivity, knowledge generation is the outcome of social constructions and translation procedures, and requires critical interrogation (Sandywell, 1996). The objective of reflexivity 'is to return human creativity to its situated sources in wider technical, political, and institutional processes' (Sandywell, 1996, p. xv), and to do so with the aim of positive possibility rather than an endless spiral of unproductive critique.

Harding (1991) elaborated on the significance of epistemic reflexivity from a feminist social justice perspective in her seminal book, *Whose Science?: Whose Knowledge?: Thinking from Women's Lives*. Harding called for reflexivity about the practices of science from the perspective of those whose voices and interests are excluded and marginalized in the production of scientific knowledge, and whose subjectivities are occluded through adoption of *a view from nowhere*. She argued that knowledge is always produced from a particular standpoint, and that claims to objectivity, in the traditional sense of the word, are not truly achievable. Harding contended that researchers must rethink objectivity in the direction of what she coined *strong objectivity*, a type of objectivity that includes reflexive attention to the subjectivities and standpoints of those who contribute to the production of knowledge, the voices excluded from the practices of knowledge production, and the practices by which knowledge is produced and used for particular ends.

Epistemic reflexivity draws attention to the epistemic cultures of a discipline, including the particular practices that create and warrant knowledge claims in a field (Knorr-Cetina, 1999). At this early stage in the evolution of occupational science, it is important to interrogate its epistemic cultures, 'those amalgams of arrangements and mechanisms . . . which, within a given field, make up *how we know what we know*' (Knorr-Cetina, 1999, p. 1). Epistemic reflexivity interrogates the practices and processes of knowledge generation, and the epistemic cultures that *legitimize* knowledge claims and inform how we know what we know. While sometimes viewed as an overwhelming process, due to the depth and complexity of issues that surface (Knorr-Cetina, 1999), epistemic reflexivity is of central concern to discussions about knowledge generation; the challenging nature of the issues arising does not constitute adequate justification for its dismissal. Epistemic reflexivity can inform occupational scientists' conscious participation in developing epistemic cultures that are responsive to the most pressing questions and problems facing the field; it can allow occupational scientists to interrogate what counts as knowledge in the discipline and to consider the values and practices that inform knowledge generation in occupational science; and it can encourage occupational scientists to consider what pluralistic approaches to knowledge generation may fruitfully contribute to scholarship in the field (Kinsella & Whiteford, 2009).

Conclusion

The seminal work of Thomas Kuhn shows how science may be viewed as a series of practices within epistemic communities. The epistemic values that individual scientists within a community weigh inform the decisions about what theories get taken up within a discipline, and the predominant knowledge paradigms within a field. Occupational scientists are members of a unique epistemic community in the early stages of development, and thus the science may be viewed as a new knowledge paradigm in its own right. The words of Thomas Kuhn (1962) are instructive:

> *If [supporters of a new paradigm] are competent, they will improve it, explore its possibilities, and show what it would be like to belong to the community guided by it. And as that goes on, if the paradigm is one destined to win its fight, the number and strength of the persuasive arguments in its favor will increase. More scientists will then be converted, and the exploration of the new paradigm will go on.* (p. 159)

The strength of occupational science is only as good as the persuasiveness of its scholarly discourse, and the quality of the conversations within its epistemic community. Occupational scientists have a responsibility to contribute to the development of their knowledge base, and to become aware of roles within this knowledge-producing community. As a new and emerging discipline occupational science is filled with epistemic promise, possibility and potential peril. While the value of technical, explanatory research is clear, it is important to listen to the many commentators who suggest that socially oriented research paradigms are also required to address complex questions in the social sciences. Many of the questions arising in occupational science fall in the realm of social science and may be best informed by approaches to research situated within interpretive and critical knowledge paradigms. Albert, Laberge, Hodges, Regehr and Lingard (2008) suggested that exposure to knowledge paradigms in the social sciences frequently contributes to broadening scientists' perspectives and to advancing more complex and pluralistic conceptions of rigour. In this chapter, I have argued for recognition of the diverse philosophical perspectives that inform knowledge generation in interpretive and critical traditions. Further explication of what unique methodologies within these traditions encompass is important work for the future of occupational science. My aim has been to advance the scientific culture within occupational science by contributing to understandings about, and calling for recognition of the philosophical foundations of pluralistic knowledge paradigms in occupational science. In addition, I have called for interrogation of the knowledge claims within occupational science through epistemic reflexivity. Finally, I have argued for conscious and collective thought within the epistemic community about the values and practices that inform the current state and future evolution of occupational science's epistemic (knowledge-producing) culture.

Acknowledgement

I am grateful to the graduate students who have participated in my philosophical foundations of qualitative research course over the last number of years, and engaged in stimulating dialogue regarding many of the topics in this chapter. Special thanks to Marie-Eve Caty for assistance in the development of Table 6.1. I also extend my appreciation to the School of Occupational Therapy and the Faculty of Health Sciences, at The University of Western Ontario, for support of this work.

References

Adorno, T. (1973). *Negative Dialectics*. London: Routledge.

Adorno, T. (1984). *Aesthetic Theory*. London: Routledge.

Albert, M., Laberge, S., Hodges, B., Regehr, G., & Lingard, L. (2008). Biomedical scientists' perception of the social sciences in health research. *Social Science and Medicine*, **66**, 2520–31.

Alexander, H. (2006). A view from somewhere: Explaining the paradigms of educational research. *Journal of Philosophy of Education*, **40**, 205–21.

Alcoff, L., & Potter, E. (1993). *Feminist Epistemologies*. London: Routledge.

Aldrich, R. (2008). From complexity theory to transactionalism: Moving occupational science forward in theorizing the complexities of behaviour. *Journal of Occupational Science*, **15**, 147–56.

Arato, A., & Gebhardt, E. (Eds). (1982). *The Essential Frankfurt School Reader*. New York: Continuum.

Argyris, C. (1994). *Knowledge for Action.* San Francisco: Jossey-Bass.
Argyris, C. Putnam, R., & Smith, D. (1985). *Action Science: Concepts, Methods and Skills for Research and Intervention.* San Francisco: Jossey-Bass.
Ashmore, M. (1989). *The Reflexive Thesis: Writing Sociology of Scientific Knowledge.* Chicago: University of Chicago Press.
Bakhtin, M. (1981). *The Dialogic Imagination* (M. Holquist, Ed.; trans. C. Emerson & M. Holquist). Austin: University of Texas Press.
Barber, M. (2006). Occupational science and the first-person perspective. *Journal of Occupational Science,* **12**, 94–6.
Benhabib, S. (1986). *Critique, Norm, and Utopia: A Study of the Foundations of Critical Theory.* New York: Columbia University Press.
Berger, P., & Luckmann, T. (1967). *The Social Construction of Reality: A Treatise on the Sociology of Knowledge.* Garden City: Anchor Books.
Bernstein, R. (2002). The constellation of hermeneutics, critical theory and deconstruction. In R.J. Dostal (Ed.), *The Cambridge Companion to Gadamer* (pp. 267–82). New York: Cambridge University Press.
Bourdieu, P. (1990). *The Logic of Practice.* Stanford: Stanford University Press. [Originally published in 1980].
Bourdieu, P. (1998). *Practical Reason: On the Theory of Action.* Stanford: Stanford University Press [Originally published in 1994].
Bourdieu, P., & Wacquant, L. (1992). *An Invitation to Reflexive Sociology.* Chicago: The University of Chicago Press.
Burr, V. (1995). *An Introduction to Social Constructionism.* New York: Routledge.
Camic, C., & Joas, H. (Eds), (2004) *The Dialogic Turn: New Roles for Sociology in a Postdisciplinary Age.* Lanham, MD: Rowman & Littlefield.
Christiansen, C., & Townsend, E. (2010). The occupational nature of social groups. In C. Christiansen & E. Townsend (Eds), *Introduction to Occupation: The Art and Science of Living* (2nd ed., pp. 175–210). Thorofare, NJ: Prentice Hall.
Code, L. (1991). *What Can She Know? Feminist Theory and the Construction of Knowledge.* Ithaca, NY: Cornell University Press.
Collins, P. (1991). *Black Feminist Thought: Knowledge, Consciousness, and the Politics of Empowerment.* New York: Routledge.
Connerton, P. (1980). *The Tragedy of Enlightenment: An Essay on the Frankfurt School.* Cambridge: Cambridge University Press.
Crotty, M. (2003). *The Foundations of Social Research: Meaning and Perspective in the Research Process.* London: Sage.
Cutchin, M., Aldrich, R., Bailliard, A., & Coppola, S. (2008). Action theories for occupational science: The contributions of Dewey and Bourdieu. *Journal of Occupational Science,* **15**, 157–65.
Darnell, R. (2002). Occupation is not a cross-cultural universal: Some reflections from an ethnographer. *Journal of Occupational Science,* **9**, 5–11.
Derrida, J. (1976). *On Grammatology.* Baltimore: Johns Hopkins University Press.
Derrida, J. (1978). *Writing and Difference.* London: Routledge & Kegan Paul.
Dewey, J. (1938). *Experience and Education.* New York: Collier Books.
Dickie, V., Cutchin, M.P., & Humphry, R. (2006). Occupation as transactional experience: A critique of individualism in occupational science. *Journal of Occupational Science,* **13**, 83–93.

Dilthey, W. (1976). The rise of hermeneutics. In P. Connerton (Ed.), *Critical Sociology: Selected Readings* (pp. 104–16). Harmondsworth: Penguin.

Dreyfus, H., & Rabinow, P. (1982). *Michel Foucault: Beyond Structuralism and Hermeneutics*. Chicago: University of Chicago Press.

Elgin, C. (1997). *Between the Absolute and the Arbitrary*. Ithaca, NY: Cornell University Press.

Feyerabend, P. (1975). *Against Method: Outline of an Anarchistic Theory of Knowledge*. London: New Left Books.

Feyerabend, P. (1993). *Against Method* (3rd ed.). London: Verso.

Fogelberg, D., & Frauwirth, S. (2010). A complexity science approach to occupation: Moving beyond the individual. *Journal of Occupational Science*, **17**, 131–9.

Foucault, M. (1972). *The Archaeology of Knowledge*. New York: Pantheon Books.

Foucault, M. (1973). *The Birth of the Clinic: An Archaeology of Medical Perception*. New York: Pantheon Books.

Foucault, M. (1980). *Power/Knowledge: Selected Interviews and Other Writings 1972–1977* (C. Gordon, Ed.; trans. D. Bouchard & S. Simon). New York: Pantheon Books.

Freire, P. (1970). *Cultural Action for Freedom*. Cambridge, MA: Centre for Study of Development and Social Change.

Freire, P. (1989). *Pedagogy of the Oppressed*. New York: Continuum.

Gadamer, H.G. (1976). *Philosophical Hermeneutics* (trans. E. Linge). Berkeley: University of California Press.

Gadamer, H.G. (1996). *Truth and Method* (2nd rev. ed.). New York: Continuum.

Gergen, K. (1994). *Realities and Relationships, Soundings in Social Construction*. Cambridge, MA: Harvard University Press.

Gergen, K. (1999). *An Invitation to Social Construction*. London: Sage.

Golinski, J. (1998). *Making Natural Knowledge: Constructivism and the History of Science*. Cambridge: Cambridge University Press.

Goodman, N. (1978). *Ways of Worldmaking*. Indianapolis: Hackett.

Goodman, N., & Elgin, C. (1988). *Reconceptualizations in Philosophy and Other Arts and Sciences*. Indianapolis: Hackett.

Gould, C. (Ed.). (2003). *Constructivism and Practice: Toward a Historical Epistemology*. New York: Rowman & Littlefield.

Gramsci, A. (1971). *The Prison Notebooks*. New York: International Publishers.

Guba, E.G., & Lincoln, Y.S. (1994). Competing paradigms in qualitative research. In N. K. Denzin & Y.S. Lincoln (Eds), *Handbook of Qualitative Research* 1st ed., pp. 105–17. Thousand Oaks, CA: Sage.

Guba, E., & Lincoln, Y. (2004). Competing paradigms in qualitative research: Theories and issues. In S. Nagy Hesse-Biber & P. Leavy (Eds), *Approaches to Qualitative Research: A Reader on Theory and Practice* (pp. 17–38). New York: Oxford University Press.

Guba, E.G., & Lincoln, Y.S. (2005). Paradigmatic controversies, contradictions, and emerging confluences. In N. Denzin & Y. Lincoln (Eds), *Handbook of Qualitative Research* (pp. 191–215). Thousand Oaks, CA: Sage.

Habermas, J. (1971). *Knowledge and Human Interests*. Boston: Beacon Press.

Habermas, J. (1974). *Theory and Practice*. London: Heinemann.

Habermas, J. (1984/1987). *The Theory of Communicative Action (Vols I & II)*. Boston: Beacon.
Hacking, I. (1999). *The Social Construction of What?* Cambridge: Harvard University Press.
Haraway, D. (1991). Situated knowledges: The science question in feminism and the privilege of partial perspective. In D. Haraway (Ed.), *Simians, Cyborgs, and Women* (pp. 138–63). Ithaca, NY: Cornell University Press.
Harding, S. (Ed.). (1987). *Feminism and Epistemology*. Bloomington, IN: Indiana University Press.
Harding, S. (1991). *Whose Science? Whose Knowledge? Thinking from Women's Lives*. Ithaca, NY: Cornell University Press.
Harding, S., & Hintikka, M. (Eds). (1983). *Discovering Reality: Feminist Perspectives on Epistemology, Metaphysics, Methodology and Philosophy of Science*. Dordrecht: Reidel Publishing.
Hegel, G. (1977). *The Phenomenology of the Spirit*. New York: Oxford Press.
Heidegger, M. (1962). *Being and Time* (trans. J. Marquarrie & E. Robinson). New York: Harper.
Heidegger, M. (1971). *On the Way to Language*. New York: Harper & Row.
Heidegger, M. (1975). *Poetry, Language, Thought*. New York: Harper Colophon.
Heidegger, M. (1977). *Basic Writings* (D.F. Krelly Ed.). New York: Harper & Row.
Hekman, S.J. (1990). *Gender and Knowledge: Elements of a Postmodern Feminism*. Cambridge, UK: Polity Press.
Hiley, D., Bohman, J., & Shusterman, R. (Eds), (1991). *The Interpretive Turn: Philosophy, Science, Culture*. Ithaca, New York: Cornell University Press.
Hocking, C. (2009). The challenge of occupation: Describing the things people do. *Journal of Occupational Science*, **16**, 140–50.
Horkheimer, M. (1982). *Critical Theory: Selected Essays*. New York: Continuum.
Horkheimer, M., & Adorno, T. (1972). *Dialectic of Enlightenment* (trans. J. Cumming). New York: Continuum.
Howe, K. (1998). The interpretive turn and the new debate in education. *Educational Researcher*, 27, 13–20.
Hoy, D.C., & McCarthy, T. (1994). *Critical Theory*. Oxford: Blackwell Publishing.
Husserl, E. (1931). *Ideas: General Introduction to Pure Phenomenology*. London: George Unwin.
Husserl, E. (1970a). *Logical Investigations (Vols I–II)*. London: Routledge & Kegan Paul.
Husserl, E. (1970b). *The Crisis of European Sciences and Transcendental Phenomenology: An Introduction to Phenomenological Philosophy* (trans. D. Carr). Bloomington, IN: Northwestern University Press.
Husserl, E. (1999). Elements of a science of the life-world. In D. Welton (Ed.), *The Essential Husserl: Basic Writings in Transcendental Phenomenology* (pp. 363–78). Bloomington, IN: Indiana University Press.
Kezar, A. (2004). Wrestling with philosophy: Improving scholarship in higher education. *The Journal of Higher Education*, 75, 42–55.
Kinsella, E.A. (2006). Hermeneutics and critical hermeneutics: Exploring possibilities within the art of interpretation. *Forum: Qualitative Social Research*, 7, Art. 19 [49 paragraphs].

Kinsella, E.A., & Whiteford, G. (2009). Knowledge generation and utilization: Toward epistemic reflexivity. *Australian Occupational Therapy Journal*, **56**, 249–58.
Knorr-Cetina, K. (1999). *Epistemic Cultures: How the Sciences Make Knowledge.* Cambridge, MA: Harvard University Press.
Kuhn, T. (1962). *The Structure of Scientific Revolutions.* Chicago: University of Chicago Press.
Kuhn, T. (1977). *The Essential Tension.* Chicago: University of Chicago Press.
Kuhn, T. (1996). *The Structure of Scientific Revolutions* (3rd ed.). Chicago: University of Chicago Press.
Kukla, A. (2000). *Social Constructivism and the Philosophy of Science.* London: Routledge.
Latour, B., & Woolgar, S. (1986) *Laboratory Life: The Construction of Scientific Facts.* Princeton: Princeton University Press.
Levinas, E. (2001). *Is it Righteous to Be?* Stanford, CA: Stanford University Press.
Lewin, K. (1951). *Field Theory in Social Science.* New York: Harper.
Lewin, K. (1997). *Resolving Social Conflicts & Field Theory in Social Science.* Washington: American Psychological Association.
Longino, H. (1990). *Science as Social Knowledge.* Princeton: Princeton University Press.
Longino, H. (2001). *The Fate of Knowledge.* Princeton: Princeton University Press.
Lyotard, J. (1979). *The Postmodern Condition: A Report on Knowledge.* Manchester: Manchester University Press.
Marx, K. (1961). *Selected Writings in Sociology and Social Philosophy* (2nd ed., T.B. Bottomore & M. Rubel Eds). Harmondsworth: Penguin. [First published in 1956].
Marx, K. (1963). *The Poverty of Philosophy.* New York: International Publishers. [Original work published in 1847].
Marx, K. (1964). *Economic and Philosophic Manuscripts of 1844.* New York: International Publishers. [Original work published in 1844].
Marx, K., & Engels, F. (1937). *The Communist Manifesto.* London: Lawrence & Wishart.
Mead, G.H. (1934). *Mind, Self and Society.* Chicago: University of Chicago Press.
Mead, G.H. (1964). *Selected Writings.* New York: Bobbs-Merrill.
Merleau-Ponty, M. (1962). *Phenomenology of Perception.* New York: Humanities Press.
Mishler, E.G. (1990). Validation in inquiry-guided research: The role of exemplars in narrative studies. *Harvard Educational Review*, **60**, 415–42.
Molineux, M., & Whiteford, G. (2006). Occupational science: Genesis, evolution and future contributions. In E. Duncan (Ed.), *Foundations for Practice in Occupational Therapy* (pp. 297–313). London: Elsevier.
Molke, D. (2009). Outlining a critical ethos for historical work in occupational science and occupational therapy. *Journal of Occupational Science*, **16**, 75–84.
Natter, W., Schatzki, T., & Jones, J. (1995). Contexts of objectivity. In W. Natter, T. Schatzki, & J. Jones (Eds), *Objectivity and its Other* (pp. 1–17). New York: Guilford Press.
Parker, I. (Ed.). (1998). *Social Constructionism, Discourse and Realism.* London: Sage.
Ponterotto, J.G. (2005). Qualitative research in counseling psychology: A primer on research paradigms and philosophy of science. *Journal of Counseling Psychology*, **52**, 126–36.

Potter, J. (1996). *Representing Reality, Discourse, Rhetoric and Social Construction.* London: Sage.

Rabinow, P., & Sullivan, W. (Eds). (1987). *Interpretive Social Science: A Second Look.* Berkeley: University of California Press.

Ralston Saul, J. (1992). *Voltaire's Bastards: The Dictatorship of Reason in the West.* Toronto: Penguin Books.

Ricoeur, P. (1974). *The Conflict of Interpretations: Essays in Hermeneutics.* Evanston: Northwestern University Press.

Ricoeur, P. (1976). *Interpretation Theory, Discourse and the Surplus of Meaning.* Fort Worth: Texas Christian University Press.

Ricoeur, P. (1981). *Hermeneutics and the Human Sciences.* Cambridge: Cambridge University Press.

Rorty, R. (1979). *Philosophy and the Mirror of Nature.* Princeton: Princeton University Press.

Rudman, D., Dennhardt, S., Fok, D. *et al.* (2008). A vision for occupational science: Reflecting on our disciplinary culture. *Journal of Occupational Science*, **15**, 136–46.

Ryle, G. (1949). *The Concept of Mind.* London: Hutchinson.

Said, E. (1978). *Orientalism.* New York: Vintage Books.

Sandywell, B. (1996). *Reflexivity and the Crisis of Western Reason: Logological Investigations*, Vol. 1. London: Routledge.

Schutz, A. (1967). *The Phenomenology of the Social World.* Chicago: University of Chicago Press.

Schutz, A. (1970). *On Phenomenology and Social Relations.* Chicago: Chicago University Press.

Shotter, J. (1993a). *Conversational Realities.* London: Sage.

Shotter, J. (1993b). *Cultural Politics of Everyday Life: Social Constructionism, Rhetoric and Knowing of the Third Kind.* Buckingham: Open University Press.

Snape, D., & Spencer, L. (2003). The foundations of qualitative research. In J. Ritchie & J. Lewis (Eds), *Qualitative Research Practice: A Guide for Social Science Students and Researchers* (pp. 1–23). Thousand Oaks, CA: Sage.

Spivak, G. (1990). *The Post-Colonial Critic: Interviews, Strategies, Dialogues.* New York: Routledge.

Stanley, L. (Ed.). (1990). *Feminist Praxis: Research, Theory and Epistemology in Feminist Sociology.* London: Routledge.

Stanley, L., & Wise, S. (1993). *Breaking Out Again: Feminist Ontology and Epistemology* (2nd ed.). London: Routledge.

Taylor, C. (1987). Interpretation and the sciences of man. In P. Rabinow & W. Sullivan (Eds), *Interpretive Social Science: A Second Look* (pp. 33–81). Berkeley: University of California Press.

Taylor, C. (1991). The dialogical self. In D. Hiley, J. Bohman & R. Shusterman (Eds), *The Interpretive Turn: Philosophy, Science and Culture* (pp. 304–14). Ithaca, NY: Cornell University Press.

Toulmin, S. (1990). *Cosmopolis: The Hidden Agenda of Modernity.* Chicago: Chicago University Press.

Weber, M. (1949). *The Methodology of the Social Sciences.* Glencoe: Free Press.

7 Occupation and ideology

Ben Sellar

Anyone who has never been obsessed by the distinction between rationality and obscurantism, between false ideology and true science, has never been modern.
Bruno Latour, 1991/1993, p. 36

Is occupational science 'modern'? Are occupational scientists opposed to ideology? It would seem that as a critical field we must stand against something and, historically, sciences have stood against ideologies. Ideology is a term of critique that is commonly invoked in one of two ways. First, we may critique someone's position as ideological, thus highlighting its prejudice, bias and narrowness in light of the objective facts. Alternatively, we might acknowledge that while we cannot escape ideology, we may still critically compare different ideologies for their relative capacity to achieve justice. While we have the option to either denounce ideology wholesale, or critique one ideology in the name of another, each critical practice relies on a form of rationality against which, or by which, to compare competing ideologies. The historical, conceptual development of ideology has bequeathed to us these two critical functions upon which occupational science has increasingly drawn as it seeks not only the determination of facts about occupation, but also the development of knowledge in support of more just and equitable societies. Such terms of critique are often found in occupational discourses where injustice is described as the failure of social, physical, institutional, or cultural environments to recognize and satisfy the occupational needs of humans (Townsend & Wilcock, 2004; Wilcock, 2006).

Occupational Science: Society, Inclusion, Participation, First Edition.
Edited by Gail Whiteford and Clare Hocking.

But the term modern, used by Latour above, is important for it implies that these binaries between rationalism and obscurantism, science and ideology are specific to a particular time, and are perhaps necessary only for a *modern* critique. In another time, whether post-modern, pre-modern, or otherwise non-modern, these terms and their relationships may be thought of differently, or perhaps dissolve entirely. In pursuit of a critical occupational science then, we may ask ourselves, 'How do we understand ideology, and might rethinking its relationship with science make possible new ways of being critical?' My argument is that a critical occupational science would pursue not only new targets for its existing critical position, but also new ways of understanding what critique can mean, and what critique can make possible.

As this chapter concerns the concept of ideology, my aim is to recast the concept in terms capable of supporting a critical capacity beyond the scope of its historical formulations. I begin with a brief discussion of the problem in occupational science and claim that the conceptual foundations on which its critical practices operate draw heavily from Marxist notions of ideology. Through a historical excursion into the theories of Marx, Engels, and Althusser, I summarize two significant approaches to the concept of ideology to show how occupational science has come to take the position it has. This allows me in the final section to attempt a redefinition of ideology in terms more adequate to the contemporary critical demands emerging in occupational science. My claim is that by seeking and embracing fresh modes of critique, occupational scientists may open new spaces for thought in which to affirm new modes of human existence.

The dichotomous ground of critique

Theories of occupational justice have drawn significantly upon the critical hinge between the world as it actually is, and the world as it is interpreted; matter and consciousness. Though rarely made explicit in either occupational science or occupational therapy, this division has served to differentiate between just and unjust social formations based on the degree of error between material reality and its representation in social organization. This position is characterized by Wilcock (2006) in her argument for an occupational perspective of health.

> *While . . . people have a natural drive to engage in occupation to meet their biological natures and needs by circumstances and design, over millennia they have constructed unjust societies that fail to recognize the needs that created them. Unless the occupational nature and needs of people are recognized in occupationally just policies, the majority of the world's population will fail to flourish.* (p. 248)

Here health is rendered as dependent upon the satisfaction of natural human needs that are separate to the historical social developments by which they have become progressively obscured. For Wilcock, while societies have changed over time, they each represent an attempt to solve the problem of how best to meet the natural needs of humans, and, whether by accident or intent, some do this better than others. Consequently, critical theory and practice towards healthier societies relies upon the advocacy for social organization that satisfies the natural drive for occupation inherent to all humans. According to Wilcock's thinking then, it seems we should turn to nature for guidance in the development of more just societies.

The importance of Wilcock's deferral to nature becomes clear when we connect it with the Universal Declaration of Human Rights (United Nations, 1948), from which occupational justice discourse draws substantial theoretical and rhetorical resources. Article 29 states that:

> *... everyone shall be subject only to such limitations as are determined by law solely for the purpose of securing due recognition and respect for the rights and freedoms of others and of meeting the just requirements of morality, public order and the general welfare in a democratic society.*

This passage highlights a complex problem for human rights. Wilcock described how social forces alienate humans from their nature and give rise to decreased health and well-being. This viewpoint underpins her argument for practitioners to take an occupational justice approach, for ill health is socially determined. At the same time though, the Universal Declaration of Human Rights advocates for the amelioration of social injustice by law, a means that is equally socially determined. From Wilcock's perspective it is social forces that have obscured our needs, but the discourse of human rights suggests that socially determined laws are necessary to secure rights and respect. If we could not defer to nature, we would arrive at a type of impasse, where social forces of liberation are deployed to address social forces of repression without any way of ensuring that the former are not in fact the latter. When we locate responsibility for historical injustice in the societies we have constructed, then a social basis for justice becomes very difficult to defend against charges of relativism, parochialism and imperialism. This is why Wilcock's invocation of natural human needs is important; they serve to relieve this tension by providing a non-social reference point for the determination of just social policy. Recognize human needs in the organization of society, and sustainable health and well-being will be your reward.

Though the political standpoint of occupational disciplines has relied strongly on this position, such a distinction between nature and society in the name of critique has been described as a practice that is particular to a time, place, and set of knowledges characteristic of modernism. This critique has been most powerfully made by Bruno Latour, a theorist in the field of science studies whose work focuses on the scientific practices by which facts are produced. Latour (1991/1993) analysed scientific laboratories as one may study a foreign culture, by taking field notes, observations and images to show the scientific processes that take messy phenomena through to clear and distinct facts. He was interested in how the products of scientific process achieve a status as persistent and universal truth denied to the products of other human practices (Harman, 2009, p. 31), and suggested that this derives in large part from a modernist concept of critique. Modernity, from this perspective, involves an attempt to purify the world through the separation of human values, societies and beliefs on one side, and objective matters of fact subject to natural laws on the other (Harman, 2009, p. 57). By purifying the world of subjectivity, locality, partiality and prejudice, the modern critic may draw closer to articulating the true conditions of reality. Thus, 'solidly grounded in the transcendental certainty of nature's laws, the modern man or woman can criticize and unveil, denounce and express indignation at irrational beliefs and unjustified dominations' (Latour, 1991/1993, p. 36). The natural ground that modern criticism provides prevents a descent into the perils of relativism, where the possibility of evaluating one social formation as more beneficial than another becomes impossible. I claim that the logics of ideology and modernity are largely coterminous and have served to provide a stable natural referent – nature – around which societies may diverge and evolve without allowing a laissez-faire politics in which 'anything goes'. They offer occupational scientists a middle ground between overt totalitarianism and social relativism where we can affirm multiculturalism by founding it upon a homogenous mono-naturalism that is the subject of scientific endeavour (Latour, 2004). But in making such critique possible, does this formulation foreclose other forms that may offer new critical directions for occupational science? By relying on a concept of nature for our critical capacity, do we quarantine it from critique, and too hastily hand responsibility for its determination to a group of scientists representative of a minority world perspective? An examination of the concept of ideology through its historical development shows how the type of critique practiced in occupational science has emerged, and where its limits lie.

Ideology through history

The inception of ideology as a concept may be traced with remarkable accuracy. Antoine Destutt de Tracy originally employed the term at the end of the eighteenth century to denote a rigorous discipline concerned with scientific analysis of the physiological laws by which ideas are produced (Eagleton, 2007, p. 64). His hope was to methodically study how physical sensations formed the building blocks of ideas so that he might establish, scientifically, the natural first principles upon which societies could develop their beliefs, and finally do away with arbitrary value positions (Festenstein & Kenny, 2005). It is ironic that in so many subsequent incarnations, ideology has come to be opposed to the very sciences that it was originally intended to serve. Indeed the historical development of this conceptual invention is characterized by fierce debate and epistemological wrestling over what ideology is, how it operates and whether it even exists, rendering any single and universal definition problematic. Eagleton outlined 16 definitions of ideology currently circulating in contemporary discourse, each with varying degrees of mutual compatibility.[1] Nevertheless, amongst such complexity particular themes may be distinguished.

Zizek (1994) charted three theoretical axes in the study of ideology, which correspond roughly to ideology as conceived in the early writings of Marx and Engels, in the thought of Althusser, and finally the later work of Marx in his magnum opus *Das Kapital*. Though each of these axes may be roughly traced to a specific historical moment they do not represent a mutually exclusive succession of chronologically distinct points along a linear continuum of conceptual development. Rather, these themes co-exist and may surface in a range of contemporary literatures. Beyond

[1] For example, many Marxist deployments of the term refer to *any* system of beliefs, while others narrow the definition to include *only* those imposed by a dominant social or political group. One cannot hold both views simultaneously without falling into contradiction.

providing a useful structure within which to explore the complex history of theoretical and political debate about the concept, this framework is instructive in showing how the critical force of ideology relies upon its mutual exclusion from science. Here I outline in greater detail the first two of Zizek's ideological axes that are particularly relevant to the exploration of the theoretical constructs on which the concept of ideology operates.[2]

Marx and Engels

Though Marx modified the concept of ideology over time, his early work in the *Economic and Philosophical Manuscripts of 1844*, *The Holy Family*, *Theses on Feuerbach* and in particular, *The German Ideology* were written in response to the philosophy of Hegel, Feuerbach and other philosophers of the period who are generally defined as idealists (Eagleton, 2007). Idealist philosophers propose that ideas exist in the mind and are, as such, quite separate from material things. They locate pure ideas in a transcendent realm that is purified from any corruption by earthly thoughts. From there they descend into the mind, and then to the body like a set of instructions or orders. Marx and Engels sought to exorcise ideas of such abstract 'purity' and to situate them within particular historical and material conditions, in order to theorize consciousness as a socially and historically produced phenomenon. From such a perspective, idealist philosophies fetishize ideas and separate them from their conditions of production, such that they come to be seen as eternal, essential, transcendent and ahistorical. While idealists hold that consciousness derives from a pure, transcendent source, Marx and Engels' theory grounds consciousness and practical action.

> *In direct contrast to German Philosophy which descends from heaven to earth, here we ascend from earth to heaven. This is to say, we do not set out from what men* [sic] *say, imagine, conceive, nor from men as narrated, thought of, imagined, conceived, in order to arrive at men in their flesh. We set out from real, active men, and on the basis of their real-life process we demonstrate the development of the ideological reflexes and echoes of this life-process ... Life is not determined by consciousness, but consciousness by life.* (Marx & Engels, 1932/1964, p. 47)

In stark contrast to the idealism of their philosophical interlocutors, Marx and Engels asserted that neither consciousness, nor the mind, nor ideas, determine how people act. Instead, the way we act composes the ideas that we have, and our actions are always socially and historically specific. Thus the critique enacted by Marx and Engels inverted the idealist position to demonstrate how ideas are produced through action.

In this formulation, ideology is conceived as a system of beliefs about a material reality that are established through interpretation. The separation of material things and the human interpretation of them is expressed above in Marx and Engels' distinction between terms of *thought* – 'imagined', 'conceived', 'narrated' and 'thought of' – and terms of

[2] Zizek's third formulation of ideology drew on Marx's later work in *Das Kapital* and in particular his concept of commodity fetishism. These developments are beyond the scope of this chapter both for their complexity, and their lack of detailed engagement by occupational science texts.

materiality – 'real', 'real-life', 'active', and 'flesh'. It is this gap between matter and meaning that is expressed in the analogy of the *camera obscura* (Marx & Engels, 1932/1964) and the concept of *false consciousness* (Engels, 1972).[3] These commonly invoked phrases suggest that, as humans, our access to material reality is mediated by our own passions and prejudices such that our image of the world may become completely inverted and give rise to an erroneous understanding of reality. From the perspective of Marx and Engels, ideologies are coherent doctrines or composite sets of beliefs and concepts that convince us of their truth, but may serve unacknowledged social or political interests (Zizek, 1994, p. 10). Representations of the material world are communicated through texts and practices in which explicit contents betray an implicit social and political motive.

Though possessed of a common-sense appeal, the establishment of a gap between reality and interpretation presents significant theoretical problems; most pressing of which is how to distinguish between oppressive ideologies that limit our freedom, and those that are emancipatory. This is similar to the problem posed earlier in the chapter regarding occupational justice and human rights. If all interpretations of reality are potentially erroneous, how can we critically compare one against another?

Such a question brings science into view because it represents a method with which to circumvent the distorting lens of ideology. Though ideology was reframed in, and eventually disappeared from Marx's later work, here it refers to 'the disconnectedness of thought from practical existence, in ways which serve objectionable political ends' (Eagleton, 2007, pp. 78–9). Ideas are ideological when disconnected from, or oblivious to their social origin. Thus Marx and Engels denounced the descent-from-heaven model espoused by the idealists as ideology par excellence, because it provides no account of how ideas are formed. What is needed is a means by which to access reality, without the biases and prejudices of power, society and history. Many Marxists claim that such a correspondence between thought and reality is possible only through scientific endeavour (Freeden, 1998). From this perspective, science is considered to be a pursuit possessed of a 'universal interest' (Aronowitz, 1988, p. 527) and is thus ideologically neutral relative to the narrow political interests of a particular social group. Emancipatory ideas may be realized only with the accurate representation of the social conditions that generate ideological illusions; this is the pursuit of science.

So, ideology and science are quite distinct in early Marxism. The former pertains to erroneous interpretation and the latter to objective discovery. Marx and Engels inverted idealism by sustaining the separation of mind and matter but reversing their causal relationship. This is not, however, the only way of conceptualizing ideology.

Althusser

The work of Louis Althusser (1970/1971) radically altered the conceptual schema of ideology by dispensing with the realm of ideas altogether and locating ideology in social practice itself. Where Marx and Engels inverted the causality of the idealists to

[3] The camera obscura was an eighteenth-century precursor to the camera and was used to produce very accurate tracings of the external environment. However, a system of mirrors was needed to correct the image's orientation as it would originally appear inverted.

show how ideas emerged from social practice to inhabit the mind, in Althusser's formulation *ideology is actually located in those practices themselves*. That is, 'an ideology always exists in an apparatus, and its practice, or practices. This existence is material' (Althusser, 1970/1971, p. 156). Ideas are not considered to take up indefinite residence in the mind following their production through social practice, but instead only exist in the practice prescribed by the apparatus and thus rely upon its repetition for their continued existence.

Locating ideology within institutional practices requires additions to Marx's classical theory of the State, but allows for a more nuanced theory of its pervasive movement through society. Althusser (1970/1971) proposed that in addition to repressive state apparatuses such as the law courts, police force and prison systems, authority is also exerted through ideological state apparatuses that include such institutions as churches, schools, and the family (pp. 136–7). What distinguishes the two types of apparatus is their mode of function. Repressive state apparatuses function predominantly by violence through the public and explicit enforcement of a legal or political mandate. Alternatively, ideological state apparatuses function by the ideological content embedded implicitly in the material practices and rituals demanded of a *good* parishioner, student, or family member. Though conceptually useful, the division between ideological and repressive functions is not this clean, as 'there is no such thing as a purely ideological apparatus' (Althusser, 1970/1971, p. 138), and thus all institutions are considered to be unique compositions of both repressive and ideological functions.

Introducing the concept of the ideological state apparatus enabled Althusser (1970/1971) to shift the notion of ideology from an intangible realm of ideas or the mind, to a modality of social relations themselves. He conceived ideological state apparatuses such as the church or school as operating through the prescription of particular rituals – in the name of redemption or education respectively – to which parishioners and students were subjected without explicit legal or disciplinary enforcement. For Althusser then, attendance at church is not the expression of a persistent, inner religious motivation, but a set of practices by which devotion is generated and maintained. For the Marxist schema, an act of prayer is an expression of inner religious beliefs that are socio-historically specific: we kneel and pray *because* we believe. In Althusser's formulation, the prayer is constitutive of ideology: we kneel and pray *in order to* believe. This departure from classical Marxist perspectives on ideology as a set of beliefs constituted by the residual and distorted perceptions of a concrete material reality is important. Far from being a secondary expression of inner ideology, here the church functions as the very mechanism that generates it (Zizek, 1994). Moreover, once the ritual has been enacted, its products do not rise to the transcendent realm of the superstructure, but remain in the material base, and therefore demand the repeated enactment of the same rituals for their continuity. Consequently, we do not act out our ideology, instead ideology acts us (Althusser, 1970/1971, pp. 162–3).

Althusser's conceptual reorientation poses some major problems that bring science back into the fold. Ideology requires a subject who will continue to repeat the practices prescribed by the apparatus. Ideology dissolves without the subject for there is no one to engage in the practices that generated and maintained it. In Althusser's text then, ideology is developed pre-consciously through the affective force of rituals prescribed by ideological structures that act to produce the subject as devoted, well educated, etc. (Eagleton, 2007, p. 148). Ideology is only made possible by the subject 'meaning, *by the category of the subject* and its functioning' (Althusser, 1970/1971, p. 160). Without someone to kneel in prayer, the ritual has no function. But this is not so for science.

Scientific discourse, in Althusser's view, has no subject because its logical propositions are true or false regardless of who holds or espouses them, and whether they are repeated or not. Scientific theories can be analysed in terms of their internal coherence and status as truth or falsehood; that is, in terms of their accuracy in relation to reality. Science is objective. But this is not to say that ideology is wrong, false or distorted as Marx suggests. Because Althusser located ideology in the realm of lived relations, it does not even qualify as knowledge, let alone non-scientific knowledge (Eagleton, 2007, p. 139). Science is a form of subjectless (see objective) knowledge where ideology (being no kind of knowledge at all) is purely subjective and located in non-theoretical material practice.

Ideology as non-science

While the complex and wide-ranging implications of these debates are beyond the scope of this chapter, it is worth noting the complexity of ideology as a concept in Althusser's text. In the early work of Marx and Engels, ideology denotes a distorted knowledge of the real world that is expressed through practice and overcome by science. Althusser repositions the concept as neither true nor false, but located within the rituals of citizenship prescribed by, and materially existent within, ideological institutions themselves. Here, ideology is to science as non-knowledge is to knowledge. Science is explicitly designated as objective, universal and ideologically neutral, while ideology is subjective and socio-historically specific.

Despite these differences, for Marx, Engels, and Althusser, science is purified of personal and political prejudice and provides access to a non-social reality. In the case of early Marxism, it is science that frees us from the deficit of personal or political prejudice and allows us to understand the real conditions by which knowledge is produced. For Althusser, science again emerges as the saviour by offering an objective knowledge that operates independently of any individual subject. Each of these formulations provides the crucial foothold for critique, because science enables us to measure a social formation against the real, material, human needs to which it should be accountable. Therefore, oppressive societies are defined as those that either fail to recognize, or actively oppress the expression of human needs while liberal societies are those that empower individuals and provide opportunities for full participation. Scientific practice thus provides access to an actual reality that is quarantined from subjective interpretation and serves as a stable reference point against which to measure the 'justness' of a given society. For over a century, the critical force of ideology has rested upon this dichotomy between nature and society, objectivity and subjectivity.

We have thus returned to the critical practice found in occupational science. By separating society from the natural occupational predispositions of the human, we are able to represent humans and their rights as a political tactic to bring about justice. We are able to oppose specific instances of social injustice by representing a more fundamental and universal human nature. This is what allows Wilcock (2006) to state that 'over millennia [humans] have constructed unjust societies that fail to recognize the needs that created them' (p. 248). This is indeed a powerful form of critique, targeted at socially produced ideologies that misrepresent nature, but it precludes nature itself from critique. We must therefore ask whether the concept of ideology rests upon a division between nature and society that is itself ideological? This question demands a redefinition of ideology, and a new articulation of what it means to be critical.

Redefining ideology

Latour (1991/1993) described the division of nature and society that underpins historical concepts of ideology as a 'modern constitution'. His language here is significant for the term constitution denotes a 'system or body of fundamental principles according to which a nation, state, or body politic is constituted and governed' (Simpson & Weiner, 1991, p. 789). That is, the critical practice that focuses upon ideology is made possible by the prior constitution of a reality that is separated into nature and society. Just as particular democratic freedoms may be ratified in a national constitution, the capacity for critique of the social in the name of the natural is sanctioned under the modern constitution. However, the latter differs insofar as the body being constituted here is not a nation, but reality itself. I will close this chapter by showing that while this constitution permits certain modes of critique, it forecloses on other ways of thinking through the problems posed by current disciplinary debates concerning justice. This final discussion will explore ways of troubling the modern constitution on which the concept of ideology rests in order to develop a renewed definition of ideology, and re-stages critique as a creative act.

The structure of the modern constitution confines politics to the side of society such that practices of governmental, institutional, and cultural negotiation are used to distinguish between those inhumane acts and those regarded as necessary for more hopeful human futures. Alternatively, on the side of nature it locates science as the practice by which we can determine the nature of our reality. Science and politics are two very distinct forms of discourse and, although contests over facts and policies occur in each, their modes of debate are quite distinct. Argument over politics takes place in courts, parliaments and policy departments. Meanwhile, negotiation over nature is contained within laboratories and field sites through a scientific discourse that demands rigour, evidence, falsifiability, and commensurability. And while we may critique society based on our knowledge of nature, there is certainly no possibility of reversing this gaze. We can and do critique bad science, for it is no better than opinion garnished by claims to impartiality, but we can never critique the subject of science itself; nature. When critical analysis is confined to the social realm, then nature is held to be beyond question.

With this perspective, let us consider the concept of the 'occupational human' that circulates in occupational science. It is typically described as a natural entity produced through the contingent historical forces of neo-Darwinian evolution and thus held to be exterior to society. The human organism resides in the realm of nature as a substance to which social meanings are later ascribed. A major issue that accompanies any such assumption that substance is the 'stuff of exteriority because if it is positioned outside analysis then its nature is beyond question' (Kirby, 2002, p. 266). Because the occupational human is situated in a non-social nature, it is subject to the investigations of science and thus absolved from analytic interrogation. This is not to imply that debates over human nature do not occur, only that they are of an order particular to the natural sciences and thus not invested with the same critical scrutiny or contest as 'social' phenomena. This critique targets the modern distinction between social forces that are available to active transformation, and natural forces available only to human interpretation and representation (Kirby, 2002). Under examination here is the modern claim that humans may be the agents of social change, but have no agency in determining their own nature, for this is the product of natural processes outside their influence. Put another way, we can affect some of the qualities attributed to the human such as rights and dignity, in their type and degree, but we cannot alter the human substance itself. As such, occupational science risks foreclosing on questions of nature, submitting them to a rationalist brand of resolution and only permitting active political debate on the issues of how best to meet its needs. When nature is cleaved from science then, the problem for political action becomes 'How best to match social conditions to natural human predispositions?'

To interrogate ideology from the political side of a reality dichotomized into nature and society would be to miss the more profound ideological operations that maintain the dichotomy itself as necessary. I argue that we must interrogate the dichotomy, as well as the processes by which it is maintained, rather than the rhetorical content of any political theory. By positing a divided reality as self-evident and necessary to justice, occupational disciplines forfeit the chance to critique those discursive forces that function to cleave nature from society in the first place. Critical immunity is achieved in one of two ways. First, the forces of dichotomization are obscured by rhetorically yolking the two halves into a bio-social holism. This move is characterized by claims that occupational science is holistic because it acknowledges both the natural and social determinants of health (Wilcock, 1993, p. 18). Second, the binary is explicitly stated as common sense and necessary in order to avoid a descent into relativism and moral paralysis. As such the modern constitution is held beyond critique precisely because it is fundamentally necessary to it. What does it mean for such a powerful conceptual formation to be implicitly or explicitly granted universal and uncontestable validity? To whom are we accountable for such conceptual developments in our own discipline? And on what terms may we critique the modern constitution, if the very possibility of critique is itself founded upon it?

Developing creative critique

This final question is somewhat discomforting and demands a clarification of terms. The word 'critical' has become overladen with modern presuppositions about the nature of ideology that haunt any attempts at its redefinition. It is therefore useful to develop new terms in which to differentiate between this modern criticality, and the type for which I am advocating here. As I have shown, the type of critique enacted under the modern constitution entails a denunciation of ideology in the name of a scientifically determined natural truth. This form of critique involves the representation of the natural as a means of stripping away false consciousness to reveal material reality. I call this 'denunciative critique', for its aim is to discredit misrepresentations of reality. If I were to simply claim that the modern constitution misrepresents 'the way things really are' I would repeat the very type of denunciative critique that I am trying to avoid. It is incumbent upon me then to describe an alternative, which I call 'creative critique' and develop it in sympathy with the concept of 'thought' proposed by Deleuze (1964/1994, 1962/2006).

A creative critique aligns itself with the philosophies of Deleuze and Nietzsche on two points: 'opposition to those whose ultimate aim is the recognition of what exists, and preference for an untimely thought which seeks to invent new possibilities for life' (Patton, 2000, p. 25). Thought, according to Deleuze (1962/2006), involves a twofold process of deconstructing established norms and values in order to create an unstructured space in which one is provoked to create new values and concepts. For Deleuze, the accurate representation of what exists is bound up in received notions of what exists that are particular to this time. As such it cannot be 'untimely thought', but timely recognition. This is not to deny that recognition occurs and has its uses, rather that recognition confines us to a space structured by established values and concepts that affords little room for these to be problematized and reinvented. Alternatively, deconstructing established values and concepts produces an indeterminate space in which the critic finds 'no-thing' to represent, and instead is provoked to inventive and creative thought. Accordingly, 'critique is destruction as joy, the aggression of the creator' (Deleuze, 1962/2006, p. 87). Destruction, or deconstruction, is a joyful act for the creative critic and involves a celebration of the possibilities for social transformation that are made possible when thought is freed from the grip of socio-historically determined truths.

A common reading of Deleuze suggests that he means to do away with all categories and deny the existence of actual things in favour of inventive thought. However, his work is more cautious than this, suggesting that thought will always actualize new categories, concepts and things (Deleuze & Guattari, 1980/2007, p. 54). When we apply thought to particular sites of contest, such as the denial of women's human rights, we are not thinking about how to defend their rights, but submitting to re-examination the conceptual categories 'woman', 'human', and 'rights' to determine what they make possible, what they prohibit, and whether their transformation would open new creative possibilities of life. This re-examination may indeed legitimate such categories and return them as politically useful, but this does not preclude them from further creative critique in the future. Ultimately, this marks a qualitative shift from the denunciative critique prescribed by the modern constitution because it demands that the critic resist invitations to the representation and defence of established concepts and values, in order to deconstruct these representations and affirm the creative act of thought.

Creative critique then may be described as the 'refusal to use concepts derived from products to discuss their own production process' (Protevi, 2001, p. 39). When analysis of a process of formation takes place on the terms of the thing thus formed, it is difficult to escape a teleological reading in which the process was destined all along to arrive at its recognizable terminal point. For example, if we take the human as given, we cannot help but read history through the moral and political values produced through socio-historically specific regimes of truth. We celebrate those ancient civilizations which – 'all that time ago' – had the insight to perceive what we now know to be 'true' about the human, such as the need for activity, the value of self-determination, and the importance of freedom to make meaning. If occupational science demands an account of human nature or humanity in order to mount critique in the name of human rights, then it risks prioritizing a human essence over perpetual human evolution. Any attempt at 'defending' the human necessarily delimits the scope of human attributes to those presently known and valued, which results in the foreclosure of other ways of rendering human history and imagining human futures. A creative critique will therefore look quite different to that made possible by Marx, Engels, Althusser, or the concept of an occupational human nature.

Butler (1993) powerfully performed such a creative critique by interrogating the political risks of settling upon a universal concept of the 'natural' human. Under the modern constitution, the potential for a phenomenon to be called into question as a political issue seems determined by its pertinence to either natural or social realms; where the former is given and the latter contestable. The questions posed, however, exemplify a creative interrogation of ideology, and a re-articulation of what it means to be political, by asking similar questions of 'nature' as one might of 'society'.[4] It is worth quoting Butler at length:

> *We might try to claim that we first know the fundamentals of the human in order to preserve and promote human life as we know it. But what if the very categories of the human have excluded those who should be described and sheltered within its terms? What if those who ought to belong to the human do not operate within the modes of reasoning and justifying validity claims that have been proffered by western forms of rationalism? Have we ever yet known the human? And what might it take to approach that knowing? Should we be wary of knowing it too soon, or any final or definitive knowing?* (p. 36)

Such questions hold the categories of science to account in a similar way to those of politics. They do not operate within the modern constitution but instead pose a serious challenge to any nature/society division and, through this subversion, appear almost nonsensical. What sense are we to make of the question, 'have we ever known the human?' for the objection may reasonably be made that we most certainly have known it. The human has been, and continues to be empirically determined through years of scientific inquiry and accumulated evidence generated through multidisciplinary experiments and trials. Yet to dismiss these questions as nonsense may serve only to reinforce the structure of denunciative critique that Butler is seeking to trouble. She is provoking a creative critique where the modern constitution no longer serves to scaffold our questions. Where occupational science may take the occupational nature of the human as our basis for critical interrogation, Butler's questions attempt to shake nature loose from its fixed foundations. Any definition of ideology as *non-scientific knowledge* no longer holds, as that would consolidate nature as impervious to interrogation.

Meillassoux (2006/2009) offered a concept of ideology adequate to the task of creative critique as outlined above by claiming that 'ideology cannot be identified with

[4] These terms are placed in quotations to acknowledge their limitations. I use them here only to show how a creative critique relates to the terms of the 'modern constitution', and not to suggest that Butler's critique relies upon them.

just any variety of deceptive representation, but is rather *any form of pseudo-rationality whose aim is to establish that what exists as a matter of fact exists necessarily* [emphasis added]' (pp. 33–4). Under such a definition, the force of Butler's questions is appreciable, for if the effect of ideology is to establish a contingent conceptual formation as *fundamentally necessary*, then the questions that subvert its necessity will be unintelligible as critique within its own terms. Thus, the questions posed by Butler above do not demand that we reposition the human within the natural order, incorporate other species under the human banner, or better establish the fundamental nature of the organism. They challenge us to reconceive of what nature is, how it is determined, who participates in this determination, who is excluded, and ultimately, what the effects of naturalizing certain knowledges may be for marginalized groups.

When ideology is no longer defined as error, and we do away with denunciation as our sole mode of critique, then critical questions need not concern right or wrong. Indeed:

> *... the question of whether or not a position is right, coherent, or interesting is, in this case, less informative than why it is we come to occupy and defend the territory that we do, what it promises us, from what it promises to protect us.* (Butler, 1995, pp. 127–8)

For occupational science to expand its critical capacity then, it must seek not only new targets for existing critical discourse, but also draw upon new understandings of what critique can mean. Such a project is important for actualizing societies that may operate outside the terms of existing categories. We might thus ask ourselves, why do we defend the notion of a natural occupational human separated from society? And, what does this promise us? Does the division between nature and society mark a more pressing target for interrogation, and provide more opportunity for social transformation than any explicitly political rhetoric? But perhaps the question of greatest critical value is, 'From what does our division of nature and society protect us?' The modern constitution protects us from relativism by fixing in place critical reference points from which to predict, anticipate and guide the future. But these points also limit critical practices to prescribed paths and preclude creative critical potentials that might disrupt existing conceptual frameworks and author as yet unanticipated futures. As a discipline we are faced with the question of whether our critique operates to preserve existing conceptual categories, or to pursue new and disruptive modes of thought. Are we deploying a historically entrenched notion of ideology to defend the modern constitution, or revising the terms of critique and embracing the constitution as a working draft?

References

Althusser, L. (1971). Ideology and ideological state apparatuses [Notes towards an investigation] (trans. B. Brewster). In *Lenin and Philosophy and Other Essays* (pp. 123–73). London: NLB. [Original work published 1970].

Aronowitz, S. (1988). The production of scientific knowledge: Science, ideology, and Marxism. In C. Nelson& L. Grossberg (Eds), *Marxism and the Interpretation of Culture* (pp. 519–37). Urbana: University of Illinois Press.

Butler, J. (1993). *Bodies that Matter: On the Discursive Limits of "Sex"*. New York: Routledge.
Butler, J. (1995). For a careful reading. In S. Benhabib, J. Butler, D. Cornell, & N. Fraser (Eds), *Feminist Contentions: A Philosophical Exchange* (pp. 127–44). New York: Routledge.
Deleuze, G. (1994). *Difference and Repetition* (trans. P. Patton). New York: Columbia University Press. [Original work published 1964].
Deleuze, G. (2006). *Nietzsche and Philosophy* (trans. H. Tomlinson). New York: Columbia University Press. [Original work published 1962].
Deleuze, G., & Guattari, F. (2007). *A Thousand Plateaus: Capitalism and Schizophrenia* (trans. B. Massumi). Minneapolis: University of Minnesota Press. [Original work published 1980].
Eagleton, T. (2007). *Ideology: An Introduction*. London: Verso.
Engels, F. (1972), Letter to Mehring. In R. Tucker (Ed.), *The Marx-Engels Reader* (2nd ed., pp. 765–7). New York: Norton.
Festenstein, M., & Kenny, M. (2005). *Political Ideologies*. Oxford: Oxford University Press.
Freeden, M. (1998). *Ideologies and Political Theory: A Conceptual Approach*. Oxford: Oxford University Press.
Harman, G. (2009). *Prince of Networks: Bruno Latour and Metaphysics*. Melbourne: re.press.
Kirby, V. (2002). When all that is solid melts into language: Judith Butler and the question of matter. *International Journal of Sexuality and Gender Studies*, 7, 265–80.
Latour, B. (1993). *We Have Never Been Modern* (trans. C. Porter). New York: Harvester Wheatsheaf. [Original work published 1991].
Latour, B. (2004). *Politics of Nature: How to Bring the Sciences into Democracy*. Cambridge, MA: Harvard University Press.
Marx, K., & Engels, F. (1964). *The German Ideology* (trans. S. Ryazanskya). Moscow: Progress Publishers. [Original work published 1932].
Meillassoux, Q. (2009). *After Finitude: An Essay on the Necessity of Contingency*. London: Continuum. [Original work published 2006].
Patton, P. (2000). *Deleuze and the Political*. London: Routledge.
Protevi, J. (2001). The organism as the judgement of God: Aristotle, Kant and Deleuze on nature (that is, on biology, theology and politics). In M. Bryden (Ed.), *Deleuze and Religion* (pp. 30–9). New York: Routledge.
Simpson, J.A., & Weiner, E.S.C. (Eds). (1991). *The Oxford English Dictionary* (2nd ed.). Oxford: Oxford University Press.
Townsend, E., & Wilcock, A. (2004). Occupational justice and client-centred practice: A dialogue in progress. *Canadian Journal of Occupational Therapy*, **71**, 75–87.
United Nations. (1948). *The Universal Declaration of Human Rights*. Retrieved 8 August 2009, from http://www.un.org/en/documents/udhr/
Wilcock, A. (1993). A theory of the human need for occupation. *Journal of Occupational Science: Australia*, **1**, 17–24.
Wilcock, A.A. (2006). *An Occupational Perspective of Health* (2nd ed.). Thorofare, NJ: Slack.
Zizek, S. (1994). *Mapping Ideology*. London: Verso.

8 Governing through occupation: Shaping expectations and possibilities

Debbie Laliberte Rudman

To address the occupational injustices and health and social inequities that are enduring features of many societies, occupational scientists must consider how complex interrelations of social, economic, political and cultural forces shape both expectations and possibilities for occupation. To support this claim, I draw on two bodies of critical social theory, critically informed life course perspectives and governmentality theory (Biggs, 2001; Holstein & Gubrium, 2000; Rose, O'Malley, & Valverde, 2006), that acknowledge that 'individual attitudes and actions do matter... but they occur within a context' (Calasanti, 2002, p. 4). In allowing that individual attitudes and actions are influential, I am rejecting an extreme structural position that conceptualizes people and their occupations as determined by external forces. Rather, I highlight approaches to studying the life course and governmentality scholarship that can expose complex contextual influences on occupation. More specifically, these theoretical approaches enable examination of how occupation is taken up within social and political processes in ways that shape expectations about the things particular types or groups of people should do. Moreover, these approaches attend to the material effects of the ways the life course and discourses come to be socially constructed. Thus, both critically informed life course perspectives and governmentality theory facilitate consideration of how processes of social organization and social control support and perpetuate policies and practices that create occupational possibilities for some people, while marginalizing, excluding or penalizing others.

I begin with an outline of the key characteristics of critical social theory, arguing that engagement with such theory will enable occupational scientists to push beyond

Occupational Science: Society, Inclusion, Participation, First Edition.
Edited by Gail Whiteford and Clare Hocking.

individualistic approaches to occupation and address the complex ways in which occupation is governed. In the second section, I discuss the heuristic value of critically informed life course perspectives for examining how social policy marks out expectations and possibilities for occupation. In the final section, work by governmentality theorists is explored for its potential to inform a broad consideration of the multitude of social authorities, social arenas and technologies at play in contemporary approaches to the government of occupation.

Engaging with critical social theory

There is a long-standing recognition within occupational science that understanding the occupational participation and engagement of individuals and collectives requires attention to context (Hocking, 2000; Yerxa *et al.*, 1989). However, recent critical analyses of occupational science have pointed to several limitations in how context has been addressed. For example, work from scholars at the University of North Carolina at Chapel Hill (see Cutchin & Dickie, Chapter 3, this volume; Cutchin *et al.*, 2008; Dickie, Cutchin, & Humphry, 2006) has pointed to the pervasiveness of an individualistic approach to the study of occupation in which contexts tend to be reified as static structures existing apart, and demanding reactions, from individuals. In addition, when contexts have been studied, the focus has largely been on the more immediate, tangible aspects, such as physical environmental features and the social networks of individuals, as opposed to macro-level political, economic or social elements (Laliberte Rudman, 2005; Whiteford, 2010).

Within the field of gerontology, there has been a similar recognition of the predominance of individualistic approaches to the study of ageing, for example, as seen in studies focused on how individuals adjust to the lifestyle challenges of retirement or how individuals accommodate to chronic disability as they age. Concern has been raised by critical gerontologists that this emphasis on individualistic approaches may perpetuate 'acquiescent functionalism' in which social problems, like poverty, isolation and workforce ageism, are attributed to individual adjustment rather than structural inequalities or economic relationships (Estes, Biggs, & Phillipson, 2003). Similarly, in occupational science, a failure to engage with theories and methodologies that consider issues of power, politics, economics and other macro-level elements may mean that the discipline has neglected the social processes and mechanisms through which occupational injustices are shaped and perpetuated.

Critical social theory provides a way forward in addressing how occupation is situated within social, cultural, political and economic contexts, and how dialectical interactions within such contexts dynamically shape the form, performance and meaning of occupation for collectives and individuals. However, defining critical social theory itself is a challenge, since this umbrella term is used to encompass a range of perspectives, such as Marxism, the work of theorists at the Frankfurt school, post-colonialism, radical feminism, queer theory, and governmentality, which both diverge and converge (Carpenter & Suto, 2008; Sayer, 2009). In this chapter, I use the term critical social theory to denote a particular approach to social research that is concerned with issues of power and justice. Critical social theory is committed to raising awareness of how injustices are socially shaped, perpetuated and practiced (Baars *et al.*, 2006; Kincheloe & McLaren, 2005). Such an approach is often characterized by an ontological position of historical or tentative realism. From this position, social reality is conceptualized as socially shaped, over time, through interactions of social, political, economic, cultural, gender and other factors in ways that particular structures and systems come to be reified. That is, such structures and systems come to be seen and experienced as natural, unchangeable and 'real'. In turn, critical social theorists seek to deconstruct perceptions of reality, particularly those aspects of structures and systems that are embedded in power relations and result in marginalization and injustice. The transformational intent of critical work involves opening up possibilities for dialogue and action regarding how practices, systems and social structures can be constructed and enacted in alternative ways that minimize human suffering and support human flourishing (Carpenter & Suto, 2008; Guba & Lincoln, 1994; Labonte *et al.*, 2005; Sayer, 2009).

A common feature of many approaches to critical social theory is that the 'way things are', or what is taken-for-granted, in a particular socio-political and historical context is taken as the starting point for problematization and deconstruction (Ainsworth & Hardy, 2004; Ballinger & Cheek, 2006; Estes *et al.*, 2003). Critical analyses attend to how such taken-for-granted views of reality are constructed through discursive and ideological means connected to power, and how particular constructions advantage some groups while simultaneously disadvantaging others (Baars *et al.*, 2006; Carpenter & Suto, 2008; Minkler & Holstein, 2008). For example, in relation to occupation, critical scholarship would seek to uncover taken-for-granted assumptions about what occupations are appropriate and should be socially supported for people in relation to age, gender, ethnicity, level of ability, citizenship status or other characteristics that pervade discourse, institutional policies and everyday practices. Rather than accept such occupational expectations and possibilities as 'natural' or 'right', such as the expectation that adult females take on the main responsibilities for caregiving of ageing parents or that skilled immigrants must re-qualify in relation to the occupational standards of receiving countries, such an approach would seek to examine how these views of reality have come to be socially constructed and circulated. It would raise questions such as: who benefits and does not benefit from the constructions; who contributes and does not contribute to the constructions; and how do the constructions contribute to inequities in relation to work, financial resources, gender relations, leisure opportunities and other realms?

Further integrating critical social theory into the study of occupation would challenge scholars to address how the negotiation, conduct and experience of occupation in everyday life is shaped within social relations of power. Starting with a definition of government as all actions designed to act upon and shape the conduct of others that align with broad political values and aims (Bennett, 2003; Rose, 1999), I use the term 'governing through occupation' to refer to the ways in which various types of social authorities shape expectations for occupation for particular individuals and collectives. Governing through occupation also encompasses the concept of occupational possibilities, which extends beyond what is expected to consider what comes to be taken-for-granted within specific socio-political contexts as ideal, ethical and 'right' occupations for particular socially constructed categories of people. In turn, this concept addresses how broader systems and structures are set up in ways that support such idealized occupations while simultaneously de-emphasizing or negatively framing other occupations (Laliberte Rudman, 2005, 2010).

Critical approaches in life course sociology

The concept of the life course, as a sequence of activities, stages and events in various life domains spanning from life to death (Mayer, 2004), has informed occupational science research both implicitly and explicitly (Francis-Connolly, 1998; Rowles, 2008; Wicks, 2005). Life course sociology has developed since the end of World War I, with changes in this field reflecting larger shifts in sociology from structural functionalist, to interpretive, constructionist and critical approaches (Mayer, 2004). Initially, the life course was treated as a naturally patterned progression of individual experience through time; for example in theories of life course development in which various ages and stages were seen as the healthy or 'normal' way to develop (Holstein & Gubrium, 2007). Critical scholarship addresses how particular constructions of the life course are formed and come to be socially interpreted as 'natural', shifting the focus to the social processes through which the life course, and the meanings assigned to it, are produced and negotiated with specific contexts. For example, Estes *et al.* (2003) raised questions regarding the political, social and cultural assumptions embedded in Erickson's theory of development, highlighting the ways in which it prioritizes productivity and uncritically incorporates and perpetuates the political, economic and patriarchal priorities of 1950s America. Baars *et al.* (2006) similarly critiqued disengagement theory which conceptualized the withdrawal of elderly people from social institutions and social relations in the 1960s as a natural part of the ageing process, pointing to how this theory served to sustain social relations and policies that marginalized seniors:

> *It is a curious logic that discovers that individuals post-65 are socially disengaged and decides that this is indicative of human nature, while ignoring the fact that their study population lived under a social regime in which age-graded retirement was a social institution. Such analyses always, and necessarily, eclipse the role of institutional power, assuming that it is nothing but an accommodation to the natural inclinations of the body. Because it deflects attention from the importance of social and political forces, naturalization can serve as a form of legitimatization of the social order.* (p. 4)

Critical approaches to the life course seek to examine the socially and historically contingent processes through which the life course is constructed. Such approaches are also concerned with how the expectations and meanings created via life course construction influence the individual negotiation of the life course, as well as the shaping of social systems and inequities (Holstein & Gubrium, 2007; Mayer, 2004). Key assumptions embedded within many critical approaches to the life course were summarized by Estes *et al.* (2003):

> *Once a particular way of constructing the life course is accepted, human ageing tends to be perceived as conforming to that model. It becomes a way of seeing that shapes*

> *what is seen, as people actively use the model as a guide for their own development. Such models become accepted by formal communities, professions and policy-makers and the collection of evidence and the formal classification of what is normal and what is deviant follows (p. 32).*

As the socially constructed life course in Western societies is often shaped in relation to what people should and should not do at particular points in life (Biggs, 2001; O'Rand, 2000), integration of critical life course perspectives into occupational science could draw attention to the ways power operates via policy, material and practical means to shape occupational expectations and possibilities. In the following sections, I outline two critically informed approaches to conceptualizing and studying the life course, and consider their applicability to the study of occupation.

Political economy, social policy and the life course

Theorists embedded in political economy focus primarily on the role of political and economic systems, and interrelated social forces, in shaping and reproducing dominant power arrangements and inequalities (Estes *et al.*, 2003). Life course work informed by political economy emphasizes the ways in which social policy operates to organize activities at a population level and, in turn, construct a particular normative life course which is supported by social institutions and programmes (Guillemard, 2005). For example, O'Rand (2000) proposed that 'social policies bear upon the organization of the life course. They influence the order, tempo, and steady or unsteady progression of social roles and transitions in the aging process' (p. 226). Such theorists seek to understand how life courses shaped through social policy and interrelated economic and political forces set out both opportunities and boundaries for individual life trajectories, including occupational participation within various life realms (Mayer, 2004).

Social policy is not viewed as a neutral tool through which social problems are addressed, but rather as a product of economic, political and social processes and forces that support and shape prevailing power arrangements and related ideological frameworks (Baars *et al.*, 2006). Social policy is analysed in relation to its material effects, in enabling the use of societal resources, including economic resources, for particular programmes and services. The symbolic effects of social policy can also be considered in relation to the creation of social spaces, institutions and systems of meaning that encourage certain forms of occupation and discourage other occupations. For example, social policies related to education create an age-graded and time-sequenced schedule of types of schools and degrees, outline what content is prioritized and excluded in curricula, set eligibility criteria that direct who is eligible for what forms of education, and determine how long engagement in particular forms of education will be financially supported by the state (Mayer, 2004). Within educational institutions, daily practices, social relations between educational authorities and students, and policies encourage preparation for and engagement in particular types of occupations, while simultaneously excluding other occupations.

In relation to the basis for exclusion, political economists have examined the ways in which particular constructions of the life course are connected to power in relation to both economic interests and gender. Within many welfare states in the Global North or

'West', social policies are seen as having played a key part in constructing and institutionalizing a threefold life course pattern tied to age norms, characterized by education during childhood and youth, work during adulthood, and retirement in old age. With the expansion of the welfare state, and the promotion of particular types of business practices and policies in a Fordist economy, this 'tripartite' life course became increasingly solidified and supported via institutional and symbolic means (Mayer, 2004). Economically, this regime prioritizes productive capacity as the organizing principle of the life course, rewarding those able to prepare for and successfully engage in the labour market, and marginalizing and penalizing those persons unable to do so (Estes *et al.*, 2003; Mayer, 2004). In relation to gender, this construction often supports and reproduces patriarchal gender relations, as various policies and programmes sustain the male breadwinner family model. Considering the combined effects of these power relations, critical feminist gerontologists point to the ways in which this life course construction, and its associated policies and programmes, shape and sustain inequities based on gender. For example, while reinforcing the reproductive roles of women, the tripartite life course is simultaneously used to support policies that create poverty for older single and widowed women who did not have consistent patterns of employment in adequate paying jobs for a sustained period due to their involvement in reproductive roles (Estes *et al.*, 2003; Minkler & Holstein, 2008).

Authors working within differential life course sociology explore the disparities resulting from dominant life course constructions within and across contexts (Mayer, 2004). As the construction of the life course is seen as resulting from power relations and struggles, such work analyses how the state regulation of the life course through social policy regulates and reproduces life chances that, in turn, create economic and health inequities (Estes *et al.*, 2003). For example, within the Canadian context, numerous occupational injustices are endured by Aboriginal peoples. In particular, despite recent improvements in overall high school completion rates, Aboriginal peoples in Canada continue to have significantly lower levels of educational achievement than non-Aboriginal Canadians at both the secondary and, in particular, post-secondary levels. Within contemporary knowledge-based economies, these inequities in education further enhance disparities in the realm of work, including higher rates of unemployment and lower average earnings (Hull, 2009). Moreover, these educational and employment disparities have been highlighted as key social determinants of the health and well-being of Aboriginal peoples in Canada (Clatworthy, 2009; Richmond, Ross, & Egeland, 2007).

Cooke (2009), informed by differential life course sociology, has situated these injustices within previous colonizing policies and programmes, such as residential schooling and the implementation of a reserve system that limited where Aboriginal people could live and what occupations they could engage in. Cooke identified the need to examine how the life course patterns of Aboriginal peoples are not supported by 'mainstream' policies and institutions, which penalize those whose lives do not conform to the normative patterns they espouse and materially support. For example, Aboriginal Canadians have higher rates of high school drop-out in the teenage years in comparison to non-Aboriginal Canadians, but also may return and subsequently complete secondary or post-secondary education later than other Canadians. This difference in the timing of education creates a cumulative pattern of disadvantage for many Aboriginal peoples, for example, associated with less continuous patterns of employment, and lower average incomes. Such disadvantages, and the resultant occupational injustices, are not inevitable or natural, but rather are shaped by a lack of policies, programmes and practices to support educational pathways that are different from the 'norm'.

Placing differential life course sociology in a global context, Calasanti (2002) examined inequalities of power relations at play in work and retirement. Calasanti's work exposed the ways in which the normative transition to retirement experienced and expected by middle-class men in the Global North requires and is supported by the lack of choice regarding leaving work experienced by many ageing workers in the Global South, regardless of health status. Calasanti argued for the need for a relational perspective when considering social policy, economic relations, equity, and life course construction that:

> *considers global and local power relations and reminds us that "pension crises" and economic insecurity in old age do not necessarily result from poor planning, but also derive from larger power structures and social relations. Whether one works, retires, or both, the experiences of each, result from individual actions within a larger social context.* (p. 17)

By considering global relations, Calasanti's (2002) work highlighted how occupational possibilities in one area of the world may be sustained through occupational injustices experienced in another area of the world. In other words, opportunities for choice in relation to occupation taken for granted in the Global North may be predicated on a sustained situation of lack of choice in the same types of occupation in the Global South, as well as for more disadvantaged groups in the Global North.

The life course as an interpretive resource: Negotiating occupation and meaning within context

Although life course scholarship informed by political economy enables consideration of the role of social policy in mapping out expectations and possibilities for occupation, it has been critiqued for incorporating a top-down deterministic notion of state power that leaves little room for individual agency (Estes *et al.*, 2003; Walker, 2006). Balanced consideration of the ways macro-level factors interact with and influence how social relations and individual lives are negotiated seems all the more important if, as many theorists contend, the traditional tripartite life course is being deinstitutionalized.

Debate regarding the extent to which the tripartite life course is being dismantled is ongoing. Nonetheless, the emergence of a post-Fordist or post-industrial life course has been proposed. This emerging post-Fordist life course has been characterized as increasingly de-standardized, non-linear and individualized, and as demanding greater individual planning, reflexivity and responsibility (Giddens, 1991; Mayer, 2004; Walker, 2006). For example, in many Western nations, entry into employment is increasingly delayed, job shifts are more common, employment interruptions due to job loss and resumed education are on the rise, and there is greater variability in the timing of retirement. These apparent changes in the life course are often celebrated, in governmental reports and popular literature, as enhancing individual flexibility and opening up a greater range of choices regarding what individuals do and when they engage in particular occupations (Guillemard, 2005). As such, changes in the life course can be analysed in relation to the occupational possibilities they open up. However, concurrently, as social policies retreat from the provision of traditional forms of welfare support, these changes are also framed as creating a new 'labyrinth of life' in which individuals are increasingly responsible for planning their occupational participation in family, work, education and other social realms. This planning also involves ensuring individual accumulation of financial, health and other required resources, and preparing for associated life course risks (Cooper, 2008; O'Rand, 2000).

Minkler and Holstein (2008) have argued that the 'individualizing of the social', referring to the re-construction of previously defined social problems into individual problems, occurring within the contemporary restructuring of the life course in many Western nations will exacerbate inequality. In relation to occupational injustices, a new set of concerns and questions arise as the possibilities for choice regarding occupation within an individualized, de-standardized life course are not evenly distributed, but are tied to health, financial and other forms of resources that are unequally distributed within particular power, structural and social relations (Laliberte Rudman, 2005; Minkler & Holstein, 2008). For example, several authors have examined the ways in which the social institution of retirement is being re-constructed in many Western countries, in line with the calls of global organizations such as the International Labour Organization and the Organization for Economic Cooperation and Development to promote active engagement of 'dependent' segments of the ageing population in the paid labour market.

Policy changes such as repealing mandatory retirement, extending the age of eligibility for public pensions, increasing financial penalties for early retirement, and decreasing the replacement value of public pensions, have been implemented to varying extents in countries in the West, justified by economic and demographic arguments (Curl & Hokenstad, 2006; Laliberte Rudman & Molke, 2009; Mann, 2007; Shuey & O'Rand, 2006). On the one hand, such policy changes may open up work opportunities for ageing individuals who wish to continue participation in this realm of occupation. However, those ageing individuals with inadequate financial resources, who are often women, persons with disabilities, or those with low levels of education, may have little choice regarding work, and may be increasingly marginalized to low paying, low skilled and unstable forms of employment (Hudson & Gonyea, 2007; Laliberte Rudman & Molke, 2009; Mann, 2007; Riach, 2007).

Life course work informed by radical constructionist perspectives seeks to examine how the life course itself is socially constructed through interactional processes, and how it is taken up and used by social groups and individuals within social relations and processes of meaning-making and identity formation. For example, rather than conceptualizing social policy as a rational governmental response to social problems, Biggs (2001), informed by the work of Bourdieu and Foucault, proposed a narrative approach to the study of social policy. For Biggs, this approach involves viewing policies as constructing and conveying stories that citizens are encouraged to live by. In relation to expectations and possibilities for occupation, Biggs asserted that social policies serve to legitimize places in which particular types of social subjects are able to negotiate publicly acceptable identities. The places highlighted in Biggs' analyses of 'positive ageing' policies in the United Kingdom in the late 1990s are intimately connected to occupation, in particular, places for work and volunteering. He raised concerns regarding the boundaries of this story, particularly for those unable or unwilling to engage in work in later life:

> *It encourages inclusion of a type that privileges work and activities that take a work-like form. As a place in which to stand and build an ageing identity, the story of later-life developed is, however, lacking. It lacks critical edge and at root, it has little place for dissident or alternative pathways for self and social development other than through work.* (p. 314)

Another example of critically informed approaches to the life course is provided by Holstein and Gubrium (2000, 2007). Informed by the work of ethnomethodologists, Berger and Luckmann, and Foucault, Holstein and Gubrium conceptualized the life course as an interpretive practice. This interpretive practice is comprised of a constellation of procedures, conditions, resources and structures of normative accountability through which everyday reality is apprehended, understood and conveyed. These authors sought to understand the 'practical activities that construct and make use of images of the life course in everyday life' (Holstein & Gubrium, 2007, p. 7). For example, they pointed to the ways in which normative ideas about what people should and should not do in relation to their stage of development inform decisions by mental health care practitioners, as well as by parents. Relating this to occupational science, the work of these authors leads to questions such as: How is the vocabulary of the life course, which names particular stages and transitions such as parenthood or job entry, and the associated norms and 'stocks of knowledge' constructed in relation to these stages and transitions used by individuals to make sense of their experiences over time?; What occupational expectations are outlined through these norms and knowledges?; How do these norms and knowledges guide the ways in which people choose and engage in occupation?; and, How is this vocabulary used by social actors in the health, legal and other systems to assess whether individuals, as evidenced by their occupational engagement, are healthy or unhealthy, normal or deviant, or eligible or ineligible for particular forms of assistance?

Governmentality scholarship and occupation

Governmentality scholarship is a growing field focused on understanding 'societal governance'; that is, the array of strategies and processes used to regulate and manage human conduct within various domains of life (Dean, 1999; Lupton, 1999). As summarized by Nadesan (2008), the key questions of concern for governmentality theorists encompass: 'How are human populations governed in contemporary societies? How is the conduct of everyday life in the family, in the school, and the workplace shaped by social relations of power? How do individuals engage in self-regulation across various contexts? How are recalcitrant or unruly individuals disciplined? How are the state, the market, and the population constituted and entwined in/through particular arts of government?' (p. 1). Within the boundaries of this chapter, a full description of the work within the field of governmentality scholarship is not feasible. Rather, particular aspects of this work that address how government involves the 'shaping of the way we act' (Dean, 2002, p. 119) are highlighted to illustrate its potential usefulness to further understanding of the diverse ways in which occupation is governed so as to align the occupational desires and choices of individuals with broader political values and aims.

Governmentality theorists build upon Foucault's work on governmentality and incorporate his conceptualization of power as intimately linked to knowledge and the production of 'truths'. Working from this basis, governmentality theorists seek to deconstruct the ways in which various social agencies and authorities, within and beyond the state, come to define particular issues as problems and attempt to guide the conduct of individuals and populations in ways embedded within, and reproductive of, broader political rationalities (Dean, 2002; Rose, O'Malley, & Valverde, 2006). Within a specific socio-historical context, power is proposed to operate in multiple sites and through multiple technologies in ways that align with, and reproduce, a specific way of thinking or political rationality.

Such a rationality addresses who and what is governed, why they should be governed, how they should be governed, and in accord with what principles and outcomes (Nadesan, 2008; Rose *et al.*). For example, work addressing childhood obesity and the governing of food consumption has addressed how school authorities and media shape the problem of childhood obesity in particular ways, and construct and promote particular family approaches to preparing, buying, managing and serving food as ideal, ethical and responsible. This work connects the particular ways occupations related to food consumption in families are being governed to broader political values and aims aligned with neoliberal political rationality,[1] related to the devolution of state responsibility, the shaping of responsible citizens and the emphasis on privatized solutions. In relation to occupational justice, it raises concerns about inattention to the societal supports and resources required to enable families to enact 'responsible', healthy food consumption, and the potential for childhood obesity to be framed within health care, education and other systems as primarily, or solely, a problem of irresponsible parenting (Henderson *et al.*, 2009; Vander Schee, 2009).

In considering contemporary approaches to government, particularly those aligned with neoliberal rationality, scholars such as Rose (1999) and Dean (1999) have emphasized that subjectivity, conceptualized as possibilities for organizing personhood, is an essential object and target of government. Thus, discourses are produced and circulated in ways that 'make up' particular kinds of ideal subjects and act upon people's sense of personal and social identity (Hacking, 1986). Such discourses promote and idealize the 'self' one should strive to be, and outline particular practices or technologies of the self as ways to work towards the ideal (Rose *et al.*, 2006).

[1] Neoliberalism, as an approach to government, while variously defined and implemented, is generally agreed to have become increasingly dominant since the late 1980s in various 'Western' nations, including Canada, Australia, United States of America, United Kingdom, and some other European nations. As a rationality, it emphasizes market logic, privatization, and 'responsible' citizenship in which individuals increasingly govern themselves (Ilcan, 2009; O'Rand, 2000).

As such, power is enacted not through top-down mechanisms of coercion, but through producing truths for people that subtly shape the ways they come to understand and act upon themselves in order to work towards self-development and fulfilment (Rose, 1999). Governmentality scholars have highlighted how discourses promoting responsible, enterprising selves have pervaded the ways in which problems and solutions have come to be framed in relation to a range of issues within many Western nations, so as to shift responsibility for previously defined social risks, such as unemployment, poverty and disability, to issues of self-care and individual responsibility (Lemke, 2001; Teghtsoonian, 2009).

As a parallel notion, in my work, I have proposed that occupation, like subjectivity, is an essential object and target of contemporary technologies of government (Laliberte Rudman, 2010). Various social authorities and agencies, such as health-care professionals, educators and workplaces, enact government via the use of technologies which shape particular occupations as possible, ideal and ethical for particular types of individuals or collectives, while simultaneously marking out other occupations as not possible, non-ideal and unethical. For example, I have been examining how discourses of retirement and retirees, circulated through Canadian media, promote particular occupations as ideal via connecting them to values and outcomes aligned with neoliberal notions of responsible citizenship.

This work, as well as that of several critical gerontologists (Mann, 2007; Riach, 2007), raises concerns regarding how these ideal occupations are being shaped and for whom such occupations are realizable. For example, consumer-based and body-management occupations, such as travelling, cosmetic surgery and physically active leisure, are often promoted within discourses of retirement as a means to achieve the ideal subjectivity of a youthful, modern, active retiree. While not negating the potential positive outcomes that could be associated with such occupations, when they are framed as 'the' ideals for later life, few positive possibilities for occupation are shaped and supported for those ageing individuals unwilling or unable to participate in such occupations due to economic, financial, health or other reasons (Laliberte Rudman, 2005; Laliberte Rudman, Huot, & Dennhardt, 2009).

Although my own work has focused on the discursive shaping of ageing and retirement within policies and media in particular Western contexts, several governmentality scholars have noted the rise of 'activation technologies' in contemporary approaches to government (Ilcan, 2009; Mann, 2007; Rose, 1999; Walters, 1997). Such technologies seek to re-make passive citizens of welfare systems, particularly those at risk of dependency, into active citizens who responsibly engage in a range of activities in order to ensure their continued self-reliance and productivity. Governmentality theory can be taken up by occupational scientists to critically question how occupation is shaped within and through such activation technologies in ways that seek to align the desires and goals of individuals and collectives with broader political aims that are not necessarily focused on well-being, equity or justice. Such research would engage with questions such as: How are ideal occupations being defined?; What occupations are particular groups of people being encouraged to take on and for what purposes?; What occupational possibilities are downplayed, excluded, or marginalized?; What rationalities underpin how ideal and non-ideal occupations are being shaped?; and Who is included and excluded in defining the ideals?

Such scholarship would add to the recent body of work in occupational science informed by critical social theory that is questioning the taken-for-granted assumptions regarding occupation held within that discipline, as well as how occupation is shaped through other social institutions. For example, Kantartzis and Molineux (Chapter 4, this volume; 2011) present a critical reflection on the current conceptualization of occupation dominant in the anglophone literature, theoretically drawing upon Berger and Luckmann, Giddens and Bourdieu to raise concerns related to power and exclusion within and through occupational science research. Another example is provided by the work of Burchett and Matheson (2010), who drew on the concept of occupational deprivation to analyse the impact of legislatively imposed restrictions on occupation, specifically policies related to prohibition from working for asylum seekers in the United Kingdom.

Conclusion

In their writings on occupational justice, Townsend and Wilcock emphasized that injustices are socially constructed (Townsend & Wilcock, 2004; Wilcock, 2005). Generating knowledge to inform approaches to address occupational injustices therefore requires attending to how injustices are shaped, often in ways that obfuscate their existence. In this chapter I have argued that engagement with critical social theory, in particular critical approaches in life course sociology and governmentality scholarship, will enable occupational scientists to more fully consider how occupations are governed in contemporary societies.

Critical social theory highlights the importance of being 'acutely aware of the context in which claims about how one ought to live are advanced' (Minkler & Holstein, 2008, p. 200). Critical analyses of how occupation is taken up politically within processes of social organization and control in ways that shape normative expectations and occupational possibilities, as well as deconstruction of taken-for-granted assumptions regarding what particular occupations should and can be engaged in, are important steps in creating the possibility for change. As articulated by Ballinger and Cheek (2006), such critical work can 'open up new opportunities: ones that can potentially embrace and celebrate more disparate, diverse and inclusive health-related practices for doing and being' (p. 216).

At the same time, a comprehensive understanding of how occupations are shaped, negotiated and experienced by individuals and collectives requires attention to not only macro-elements of contexts, but also individual lives. As stated by Baars (2006):

> *The structural approach cannot deduct from its analysis how specific circumstances are experienced by the persons living through them; here a narrative approach has a better chance. But the narrative perspective cannot clarify how the circumstances that are shown in the narratives as generating problems are produced and how they can be structurally improved. Both paradigms have their own indispensible value.* (p. 39)

One way to link structural and narrative approaches, suggested by Gubrium and Holstein (1998, 2009), that I am currently taking on within my own work involves examining ways in which discourses pertaining to occupation are used as interpretive resources by individuals as they construct narratives about who they are and what they do. Further dialogue within occupational science regarding theoretical and methodological approaches to considering the interplay between macro-level contextual features and the enactment and experience of occupation by collectives and individuals would further enhance the capacity of scholars to address occupational injustices.

Moreover, deconstruction, as a central element of work informed by critical social theory, is not an end in and of itself. In his discussion of the contemporary limits of critical social theory, Sayer (2009) argued that deconstruction, or the reduction of illusion, is not sufficient as it does not necessarily identify 'what things "are not right as they are", and why' (p. 781). Articulating such a standpoint on why things are not 'right', in turn, means that researchers need to attend to the political nature of their work and articulate the conception of well-being or 'justice' which informs their critique (Sayer). Labonte *et al.* (2005) similarly argued that critical population health researchers must explicate the moral and ethical underpinnings of their work, proposing that:

> *Morality without evidence risks righteousness; evidence without a moral base risks passivity. A critical approach to population health research, then, is a rare opportunity where the moral and political necessities for social change can become part of our daily work, as much a statement of who we are as of what we do.* (p. 15)

In considering the transformative potential of critical work in occupational science, it is therefore important to consider what are the 'ethics of action' (Rylko-Bauer, Singer, & Willigen, 2006) that underlie our work, both as individuals and as members of the discipline of occupational science: What rights do we see as imperative for all people? What values do we seek to enact? How are we conceptualizing 'justice'? As such, engagement in critical work demands ongoing critical reflexivity regarding our own work and transparency regarding its underpinnings.

References

Ainsworth, S., & Hardy, C. (2004). Critical discourse analysis and identity: Why bother? *Critical Discourse Studies*, **1**, 225–59.

Baars, J. (2006). Beyond neomodernism, antimodernism, and postmodernism: Basic categories for contemporary critical gerontology. In J. Baars, D. Dannefer, C. Phillipson, & A. Walker (Eds), *Aging, Globalization and Inequality: The New Critical Gerontology* (pp. 17–42). New York: Baywood.

Baars, J., Dannefer, D., Phillipson, C., & Walker, A. (2006). Critical perspectives in social gerontology. In J. Baars, D. Dannefer, C. Phillipson, & A. Walker (Eds), *Aging, Globalization and Inequality: The New Critical Gerontology* (pp. 1–14). New York: Baywood.

Ballinger, C., & Cheek, J. (2006). Discourse analysis in action: The construction of risk in a community day hospital. In L. Finlay & C. Ballinger (Eds), *Qualitative Research for Allied Health Professionals: Challenging Choices* (pp. 200–17). Chichester, England: John Wiley & Sons, Ltd.

Bennett, T. (2003). Culture and governmentality. In J.Z. Bratich, J. Packer, & C. McCarthy (Eds), *Foucault, Cultural Studies and Governmentality* (pp. 47–66). Albany, NY: State University of New York Press.

Biggs, S. (2001). Toward critical narrativity: Stories of aging in contemporary social policy. *Journal of Aging Studies*, **15**, 303–16.

Burchett, N., & Matheson, R. (2010). The need for belonging: The impact of restrictions on working on the well-being of an asylum seeker. *Journal of Occupational Science*, **17**, 85–91.

Calasanti, T. (2002). Work and retirement in the 21st century: Integrating issues of diversity and globalization. *Ageing International*, **27**, 3–20.

Carpenter, C., & Suto, M. (2008). *Qualitative Research for Occupational and Physical Therapists: A Practical Guide*. Oxford: Blackwell Publishing.

Clatworthy, S. (2009). Some estimates of private and social benefits of improving educational attainment among Registered Indian youth and young adults. In J.P. White, D. Beavon, J. Peters, & N. Spence (Eds), *Aboriginal Education: Current Crisis and Future Alternatives* (pp. 321–62). Toronto: Thomson Educational.

Cooke, M. (2009). Taking a life course perspective in Aboriginal policy research. *Canadian Issues*, Winter, 5–9.

Cooper, M. (2008). The inequality of security: Winners and losers in the risk society. *Human Relations*, **61**, 1229–58.

Curl, A.L., & Hokenstad, M.C.T. (2006). Reshaping retirement policies in post-industrial nations: The need for flexibility. *Journal of Sociology & Social Welfare*, **23**, 85–106.

Cutchin, M.P., Aldrich, R.M., Balliard, A.L., & Coppola, S. (2008). Action theories for occupational science: The contributions of Dewey and Bourdieu. *Journal of Occupational Science*, **15**, 157–65.

Dean, M. (1999). Risk, calculable and incalculable. In D. Lupton (Ed.), *Risk and Sociocultural Theory: New Directions and Perspectives* (pp. 131–59). Cambridge: Cambridge University Press.

Dean, M. (2002). Powers of life and death beyond governmentality. *Cultural Values*, **6**, 119–38.

Dickie, V., Cutchin, M.P., & Humphry, R. (2006). Occupation as transactional experience: A critique of individualism in occupational science. *Journal of Occupational Science*, **13**, 83–93.

Estes, C.L., Biggs, S., & Phillipson, C. (2003). *Social Theory, Social Policy and Ageing: A Critical Introduction*. Berkshire, England: Open University Press.

Francis-Connolly, E. (1998). It never ends: Mothering as a lifetime occupation. *Scandinavian Journal of Occupational Therapy*, **5**, 149–55.

Giddens, A. (1991). *Modernity and Self-identity: Self and Society in the Late Modern Age*. Stanford, CA: Stanford University Press.

Guba, E.G., & Lincoln, Y.S. (1994). Competing paradigms in qualitative research. In N.K. Denzin & Y.S. Lincoln (Eds), *Handbook of Qualitative Research* (1st ed., pp. 105–17). Thousand Oaks, CA: Sage.

Gubrium, J.F., & Holstein, J.A. (1998). Narrative practice and the coherence of personal stories. *The Sociological Quarterly*, **39**, 163–87.

Gubrium, J.F., & Holstein, J.A. (2009). *Analyzing Narrative Reality*. Thousand Oaks, CA: Sage.

Guillemard, A. (2005). The advent of a flexible life-course and the reconfiguration of welfare. In J.G. Andersen, A.M. Guillemard, P.H. Jensen, & B. Pfau-Effinger (Eds), *The Changing Face of Welfare* (pp. 55–76). Bristol: Policy Press.

Hacking, I. (1986). Making up people. In T.C. Heller, M. Sosna & D.E. Wellbery (Eds), *Reconstructing Individualism* (pp. 222–36). Stanford: Stanford University Press.

Henderson, J., Coveney, J., Ward, P., & Taylor, A. (2009). Governing childhood obesity: Framing regulation of fast food advertising in the Australian print media. *Social Science & Medicine*, **69**, 1402–8.

Hocking, C. (2000). Occupational science: A stock take of accumulated insights. *Journal of Occupational Science*, **7**, 61–7.

Holstein, J.A., & Gubrium, J.F. (2000). *Constructing the Life Course* (2nd ed.). New York: General Hall.

Holstein, J.A., & Gubrium, J. F. (2007). Constructionist perspectives on the life course. *Sociology Compass*, **1**, 1–18.

Hudson, R.B., & Gonyea, J.G. (2007). The evolving role of public policy in promoting work and retirement. *Generations*, **31**, 68–75.

Hull, J. (2009). Aboriginal youth, education and labour market outcomes. In J.P. White, D. Beavon, J. Peters, & N. Spence (Eds), *Aboriginal Education: Current Crisis and Future Alternatives* (pp. 309–20). Toronto: Thomson Educational.

Ilcan, S. (2009). Privatizing responsibility: Public sector reform under neoliberal government. *Canadian Review of Sociology*, **46**, 207–34.

Kantartzis, S., & Molineux, M. (2011). The influence of Western society's construction of a healthy daily life on the conceptualisation of occupation. *Journal of Occupational Science*, **18**, 62–80.

Kincheloe, J.L., & McLaren, P. (2005). Rethinking critical theory and qualitative research. In M. K. Denzin & Y.S. Lincoln (Eds), *Handbook of Qualitative Research* (3rd ed., pp. 303–42). Thousand Oaks, CA: Sage.

Labonte, R., Polanyi, M., Muhajarine, N., McIntosh, T., & Williams, A. (2005). Beyond the divides: Towards critical population health research. *Critical Public Health*, **15**, 5–17.

Laliberte Rudman, D. (2005). Understanding political influences on occupational possibilities. *Journal of Occupational Science*, **12**, 149–60.

Laliberte Rudman, D. (2010). Occupational possibilities. *Journal of Occupational Science*, **17**, 55–9.

Laliberte Rudman, D., Huot, S., & Dennhardt, S. (2009). Shaping ideal places for retirement: Occupational possibilities within contemporary media. *Journal of Occupational Science*, **16**, 18–24.

Laliberte Rudman, D., & Molke, D. (2009). Forever productive: The discursive shaping of later life workers in contemporary Canadian media. *Work*, **32**, 377–89.

Lemke, T. (2001). The birth of biopolitics: Michel Foucault's lecture at the College de France on neo-liberal governmentality. *Economy & Society*, **30**, 190–207.

Lupton, D. (1999). Introduction: Risk and sociocultural theory. In D. Lupton (Ed.), *Risk and Sociocultural Theory: New Directions and Perspectives* (pp. 1–11). Cambridge: Cambridge University Press.

Mann, K. (2007). Activation, retirement planning and restraining the 'third age'. *Social Policy & Society*, **6**, 279–92.
Mayer, K.U. (2004). Whose lives? How history, societies and institutions define and shape life courses. *Research in Human Development*, **1**, 161–87.
Minkler, M., & Holstein, M.B. (2008). From civil rights to… civic engagement? Concerns of two older critical gerontologists about a 'new social movement' and what it portends. *Journal of Aging Studies*, **22**, 196–204.
Nadesan, M.H. (2008). *Governmentality, Biopower and Everyday Life*. New York: Routledge.
O'Rand, A.M. (2000). Risk, rationality and modernity: Social policy and the aging self. In K. Warner Schaie, & J. Hendricks (Eds), *The Evolution of the Aging Self: The Societal Impact on the Aging Process* (pp. 225–47). New York: Springer.
Riach, K. (2007). 'Othering' older worker identity in recruitment. *Human Relations*, **60**, 1701–26.
Richmond, C., Ross, N.A., & Egeland, G.M. (2007). Societal resources and thriving health: A new approach for understanding the health of Indigenous Canadians. *American Journal of Public Health*, **97**, 1827–33.
Rose, N. (1999). *Powers of Freedom: Reframing Political Thought*. Cambridge: University of Cambridge Press.
Rose, N., O'Malley, P., & Valverde, M. (2006). Governmentality. *Annual Review of Law and Social Science*, **2**, 83–104.
Rowles, G.D. (2008). Place in occupational science: A life course perspective on the role of environmental context in the quest for meaning. *Journal of Occupational Science*, **15**, 127–35.
Rylko-Bauer, B., Singer, M., & Willigen, J. (2006). Reclaiming applied anthropology: Its past, present and future. *American Anthropologist*, **108**, 178–90.
Sayer, A. (2009). Who's afraid of critical social science? *Current Sociology*, **57**, 767–86.
Shuey, K.M., & O'Rand, A.M. (2006). Changing demographics and new pension risks. *Research on Aging*, **3**, 317–40.
Teghtsoonian, K. (2009). Depression and mental health in neoliberal times: A critical analysis of policy and discourse. *Social Science & Medicine*, **69**, 28–35.
Townsend, E., & Wilcock, A.A. (2004). Occupational justice. In C.H. Christiansen & E.A. Townsend (Eds), *Introduction to Occupation: The Art and Science of Living* (pp. 243–73). Thorofare, NJ: Prentice Hall.
Vander Schee, C. (2009). Fruit, vegetables, fatness and Foucault: Governing students and their families through school health policy. *Journal of Education Policy*, **24**, 557–74.
Walker, A. (2006). Reexamining the political economy of aging: Understanding the structure/agency tension. In J. Baars, D. Dannefer, C. Phillipson, & A. Walker (Eds), *Aging, Globalization and Inequality: The New Critical Gerontology* (pp. 59–80). New York: Baywood.
Walters, W. (1997). The 'active society': New designs for social policy. *Policy and Politics*, **25**, 231–4.
Whiteford, G. (2010). Occupation in context. In M. Curtin, M. Molineux, & J. Supyk-Mellson (Eds), *Occupational Therapy and Physical Dysfunction – Enabling Occupation* (6th ed., pp. 135–49). London: Elsevier.

Wicks, A. (2005). Understanding occupational potential. *Journal of Occupational Science*, **12**, 130–9.

Wilcock, A.A. (2005). Older people and occupational justice. In A. McIntyre & A. Atwal (Eds), *Occupational Therapy and Older People* (pp. 14–26). Oxford: Blackwell Publishing.

Yerxa, E.J., Clark, F., Frank, G. *et al.* (1989). *Occupational Science: The Foundation for New Models of Practice*. New York: Haworth Press.

9

When occupation goes 'wrong': A critical reflection on risk discourses and their relevance in shaping occupation

Silke Dennhardt and Debbie Laliberte Rudman

Risk has become a pervasive part of contemporary Western society. Every day, people encounter many risk-related messages in pursuing their occupations. It has become almost impossible to avoid risk-related messages associated with objects used to engage in occupations and the contexts in which occupations are carried out; indeed, references to risk have become a taken-for-granted part of modern everyday life. For example, when making breakfast, food labels bear reminders to not pursue this occupation thoughtlessly, but rather to employ it to combat future health risks. Every breakfast can become a 'smart start' in the quest for a long, healthy and disease-free life as it provides the chance to 'make our heart *one bowl* stronger' (Kellogg's Smart Start®, 2011). Food products with names like Praeventia (Praeventia Bars, 2011) or On Track Cereal (President's Choice On Track Cereal, 2011) encourage people to include preventive thinking in their daily occupations, provide reassurance about being 'on track' to maximizing their lives and validate an epidemiological mindset that 'life is a process of selecting a cause of death' (Levin, cited in JECH.com, 2005, p. 1103). Contexts for occupations have also been re-shaped by risk discourses. For example, while a common narrative of many middle-class adults in North America is that they pursued a wide range of unsupervised, spontaneous and often excitingly risky occupations in their neighbourhoods as children, their own children engage in

Occupational Science: Society, Inclusion, Participation, First Edition.
Edited by Gail Whiteford and Clare Hocking.

occupation differently. Recurrently rationalized by increasing risks, today's childhood occupations in North America are increasingly pre-planned, organized and supervised (O'Brien & Smith, 2002).

Scholars have proposed that in contemporary risk-averse society (Beck, 1992; Furedi, 2006; Gill, 2007) many things, such as obesity, genes and lifestyles, become 'risks', hence framed as predictable, preventable and controllable. Within and through risk discourses, critical health and social issues are re-framed, new practices are promoted, and new social realities are shaped. For example, in particular contexts 'accidents' gradually disappear, intentionally replaced by the term 'preventable injuries', which in turn frames how such injuries are thought of and what is done in relation to them. At their workplace, individuals learn that 'there are really *no accidents*' (Workplace Safety & Insurance Board Ontario, 2008, p. 4) as prevention strategies are available, and the editors of one scientific journal proudly announced that they had 'banned' the word accident from their journal as 'accidents are not unpredictable' (Davis & Pless, 2001, p. 1320). Such transformations raise questions about the social consequences that risk discourses have in re-shaping realities of social life, particularly occupation. For instance, who is deemed responsible (and financially accountable) when workplace or school occupations go 'wrong' because individuals 'failed' to envision the risks involved, or simply did not have the means to perform these occupations in recommended risk-reducing ways?

In this chapter, we argue that risk is a highly relevant topic and a beneficial theoretical lens to extend knowledge about human occupation beyond the individual level. We call upon occupational scientists to critically reflect on the various ways in which risk is conceptualized, and the implications of such conceptualizations for how risk is thought of and studied in relation to occupation. By introducing four major approaches to risk, we argue that it is necessary to strengthen the use of particular, critically oriented epistemologies when studying risk and occupation. Such critically informed work would consider how what is thought of and researched as a 'risk' shapes what comes to be seen as healthy, responsible, ethical or desirable occupations for particular types or categories of people. As risk is not an inherently neutral concept, but rather is based on moral and cultural values of those with power to define risks (Slovic, 1999), it is crucial to consider how risk is and can be conceptualized and related to occupation.

In addition to the contemporary pervasiveness of risk discourses, there is another reason why risk is relevant to occupational scientists. While discussions about the nature of risk and its effects on people's everyday life have emerged in various disciplines, including medicine, public health, sociology, psychology, law and economics, there is no consensus on how risk should be defined.[1] However, and intriguingly for occupational science, most risk definitions are based on the idea that humans can (and should) control their future *through their activities* (Zinn, 2008). Once a risk is outlined discourses urge individuals 'to *do* something' about it, such as, to avoid, decide for, alter, or engage in a particular behaviour or activity to manage uncertainty and minimize risk. If the future were considered as predetermined or independent of human activities, the term 'risk' would make no sense at all (Renn, 1992). This frequent and strong link to *doing* inherent in risk conceptualizations makes risk a vital focus for investigation in occupational science. However, despite its strong link to human activity, an explicit, critical discussion about

[1] Furthermore, as this chapter will illustrate, trying to reach such an agreement would be meaningless due to key differences in the epistemological underpinnings of various risk conceptualizations.

Table 9.1 Risk definitions and theoretical perspectives

Name	Epistemology	Ontology	Major theorists	Potential research foci for occupational science
Technico-scientific	Realist	• Risk is an objective phenomenon that can be measured, identified and calculated • Risk exists independently of social-cultural processes, although they can bias the perception of risk	Multiple, no specific one	What risks to humans are associated with specific occupations? How should risks related to an individual's occupations be assessed and managed? How can individuals be encouraged to make occupational choices that reduce risks?
Risk society	Weak constructionist	• Objective risks exist, but knowledge about risks is influenced by social-cultural-political processes • Many risks are 'man-made', they are unleashed by modernity's unlimited drive for progression • Risk represents a meta-narrative of our times; we live in an age of 'manufactured uncertainty'	Beck (1992) Giddens (1990)	What is the relationship of risk and occupation in late modernity? How does the breakdown of securities related to one's occupations within processes of de-traditionalization and individualization influence how people convey and construct their occupational identities? How does living in a risk society shape one's occupational repertoire?
Cultural/symbolic	Weak constructionist	• Risks are socially selected and constructed • What is selected as a risk is influenced by a group's social structure • Risks are a means to ensure social and individual boundaries	Douglas (1992)	Why are some occupations selected as risky and others not? How does risk function in maintaining and conveying a group's values – such as health – through occupations? How is risk utilized to blame people who pursue occupations that are 'other' than the normative? What is the social context in which particular occupations become valued as 'risky' or 'safe'?

(continued)

Table 9.1 (*Continued*)

Name	Epistemology	Ontology	Major theorists	Potential research foci for occupational science
Govern-mentality	Strong constructionist	• Risks are a fully human construction, they are a product of historical, social and political processes • Risk is mobilized as a technique to govern individuals, which attempts to shape rational, responsible and independent citizens	Castel (1991) Dean (2010) Ericson (1997) Ewald (1991) O'Malley (2000) Rose (1999)	How do discourses about risk and related practices operate in the construction of subjectivity and social life through occupation? Who benefits by encouraging individuals to make particular occupational choices framed as responsible 'in the name of risk'? How have risks and occupations come to be constructed differently in varying political contexts or across historical times?

Source: Adapted from Lupton, 1999a, p. 35.

risk, and its potential influence on what people do and are expected to do, is absent within occupational science literature.

Moreover, how occupational scientists as researchers, scholars and activists understand risk and relate it to occupation simultaneously frames problems, possible actions and proposed solutions (Hilgartner, 1985). It informs actions, such as the questions that are considered important to ask, the knowledge practices that identify specific populations as at-risk, or the activities proposed as the best ways to address risks. In this sense, the conceptualization of risk is inherently connected to power (Slovic, 1999), which points to the necessity of critical reflexivity regarding the ways risk is defined in occupational science:

> *Whoever controls the definition of risk controls the rational solution to the problem at hand. If risk is defined one way, then one option will rise to the top as the most cost-effective or the safest or the best. If it is defined another way, perhaps incorporating qualitative characteristics and other contextual factors, one will likely get a different ordering of action solutions. Defining risk is thus an exercise in power.* (Slovic, 1999, p. 689)

Mapping risk

The work of Deborah Lupton (1999a, 1999b), which highlights differences in underlying knowledge paradigms,[2] illustrates the diversity of epistemological perspectives on risk. Lupton (1999a) outlined four major perspectives along an epistemological continuum: Technico-scientific, Risk society, Cultural/symbolic, and Governmentality (see Table 9.1). Placing the technico-scientific perspective on a realist pole, as it focuses on risk as an objective hazard, Lupton grouped the other three perspectives as sociocultural perspectives, as they all focus on risk as relative and socially constructed to varying degrees. Within this chapter, these four perspectives on risk are summarized and their implications for the study of occupation are explored.

Technico-scientific perspective

The *technico-scientific* perspective on risk has been dominant in many fields, although studies which employ this perspective rarely define risk or explicitly address epistemology. In line with a realist position, its key ontological assumption is that risk just 'is'; that is, risk is understood as an objective, neutral entity that pre-exists 'out there', independently from humans and their perception of risk. In turn, generating knowledge about risk is viewed as a technical, value-neutral matter achieved through empirical, scientific research. Such research aims to identify and measure risk and its properties and determinants, in order to predict and control risks and develop evidence-based interventions. Therefore, from a *technico-scientific* perspective, risk is simply defined as 'the product of the probability and consequences (magnitude and severity) of an adverse effect' (Bradbury, 1989, p. 382).

[2] For epistemological stances and knowledge paradigms, see Kinsella, 'Knowledge paradigms in occupational science: Pluralistic perspectives' in this volume.

As risk is proposed to be objective and separated from value systems, its existence in this perspective is generally beyond debate (O'Byrne & Holmes, 2007). However, what are debatable are the appropriate means to measure, calculate and subsequently manage identified risks. A key aim within the technico-scientific perspective is to optimize the accuracy and techniques of risk assessment to determine the risks of, for example, engaging or not engaging in a particular behaviour. By doing so, technico-scientific researchers produce 'webs of causality' (Petersen & Lupton, 1996), which are translated into risk-reduction recommendations. Of particular interest to occupational science is that much of this research, and subsequent recommendations, pertain to everyday occupations; for example, research on reducing risks associated with work-related occupations or managing bodily risks through physically oriented occupations.

A technico-scientific perspective on risk works from a particular hierarchy of knowledge in which subjective (lay) appraisals of risk are viewed as subordinate to objective (expert) assessments and measurements of risk (Douglas, 1990; Lupton, 1999a; Slovic, 1999). This hierarchy stems from an underlying assumption that lay individuals do not possess sufficient or 'true' information as they are easily biased by subjective perceptions, experiences and values. This creates a need for experts to utilize value-free means of understanding and intervening. Consequently, there is a strong emphasis on bringing scientific knowledge into people's everyday lives by bridging knowledge gaps, stressing 'risk communication' or 'knowledge translation'. In such translation activities, human beings are often assumed to be rational actors, or 'information-processing units', who value knowledge gained through scientific methods and act accordingly (Lupton, 1999a). For example, it is expected that rational individuals aim to minimize health risks by pursing occupations proposed by experts as healthy (such as physical occupations) while avoiding occupations associated with poor health (such as sedentary occupations). If behavioural change in the face of identified risks is absent, the problem is most often assumed to be related to knowledge acquisition or transformation processes. Thus, the technico-scientific perspective on risk works on a linear relationship: once a risk is identified and truly 'understood', there is a universal rational way to act that decreases risks. Since rational individuals strive to adopt practices that prevent risks, the epistemological imperative is to uncover existing relationships between particular risks and specific activities, and to promote integration of risk-reduction practices into everyday life.

Occupational scientists who take a technico-scientific perspective might research risks associated with specific occupations, the absence of specific occupations, or an imbalance between specific types of occupations. Researchers might study how specific populations, such as 'obese children' or 'frail elderly', identified as being 'at-risk' can optimize, balance, or adapt their occupations to reduce health risks, or how individuals can be encouraged to make occupational choices that prevent risks.

The technico-scientific perspective has been critiqued for its underlying assumption of risk as being 'out there', independent from human activity and perception. Even when based on realist ontology, some risks have to be understood as, constructed, in a basic technical sense of the term (Adam, Beck, & Van Loon, 2000). For example, risks related to genetic technology did not exist previously; rather, they were constructed within a network of socially, politically and culturally located factors (Beck, 1992; Giddens, 1990). Another key critique is the perspective's underlying ideal of individuals as independent, rational actors who predominantly act (or should act) based on knowledge, independent from socio-cultural and historical-political contexts (Douglas, 1990; Rose, 1999).

Risk Society Perspective

First introduced by the German sociologist Beck (1992), the risk society perspective has also been contributed to by Giddens (1990, 1991), a British sociologist. Both theorists conceptualize risk as fundamental to the development of late modernity and its emergent social order (Jaeger, 2001), and address transformations and experiences of risk within processes of modernization. Beck (1992) argued that contemporary Western societies have entered a transitional period in which industrial society is becoming a 'risk society'. While industrial modernity was characterized by confidence in the possibility of safety, security, predictability, and the stability of traditional social categories (based on class, gender, work, or locality), risk society is characterized by an all-embracing insecurity generated by uncontrollable risks, manufactured uncertainties, and processes of de-traditionalization. Fuelled by an ongoing drive for unlimited progress and rationalization, risks emerge as unanticipated 'side-effects' of modernization processes. Therefore risk, in this perspective, is understood as '*a systematic way of dealing with hazards and insecurities induced and introduced by modernization itself*' (Beck, 1992, p. 21, original emphasis).

Beck argued that the growing focus on risk in everyday life occurs not because the quantity of risks has increased, but rather, because of the 'de-bounding' of a new type and quality of uncontrollable risks. While Beck's early work was critiqued for being inconsistent in the ontological position on 'risk' that he articulated in later works, he adopts both a realist and constructionist perspective on risk (Beck, 1999), arguing that the common distinction between nature and culture (i.e., between realism and constructivism) is an idea of modernity itself and that the two cannot be separated. Thus, while risks are viewed as socially constructed through specific measurement and assessment techniques, socially constructed risks have at the same time real lasting effects on individuals and society (Beck, 1999; Zinn, 2008).

The risk society perspective proposes that modernization processes are undermining the ontological security[3] of humans and enhancing uncertainty in two different, but interlinked, ways. First, modernization has produced a *new type and quality of risks*, essentially different from risks faced in earlier periods. Key to this, these new types of risks – such as nuclear, chemical, ecological and genetic risks – is that they transgress spatial, temporal and social boundaries (Beck, 2002). Most of them are also invisible and irreversible. For example, the risks of genetic engineering cannot be limited by time, place or class: they might affect future generations, cross contemporary geopolitical boundaries, go beyond an accountability based on established rules of causality and liability, and are impossible to insure or compensate against (Beck, 1999).

Second, modernization is associated with individualization processes that produce insecurities and new risks related to the configuration of individual biographies, life

[3] Giddens (1990) defined 'ontological security' as 'the confidence that most human beings have in the continuity of their self-identity and in the constancy of the surrounding social and material environments of *action*' (p. 92, emphasis added).

transitions and formations of identity. As traditional social and institutional structures such as class, gender, work and locality become progressively weakened, individual life becomes less certain. Such transformations lead to a categorical shift between the individual and society; it is now the individual who becomes the 'reproduction unit for the social in the lifeworld' (Beck, 1992, p. 130). An individual's biography, once understood as largely socially prescribed, becomes viewed as reflexively self-produced. It becomes a 'do-it-yourself biography' (Beck, 1992), a 'planning project' (Beck-Gernsheim, 1996), in which potential risks need to be proactively minimized. Within such individualization processes, unfortunate events, such as unemployment or chronic illness, become transformed into personal failures, rather than being considered as societal problems (Beck, 1992).

Occupational scientists who draw on the risk society perspective and consider theoretical ideas regarding reflexive modernization might study the specific relationship of risk and occupation in late modernity. For example, forefronting the breakdown of ontological securities and life course expectations within processes of de-traditionalization and individualization, occupational scientists might research how individuals convey and construct their occupations and occupational identities in times of uncertainty. As well, occupational scientists might address the implications of the increasing demands to be reflexive and proactive for occupational possibilities; for example, examining the implications for increasing demands to plan ahead for one's child's future through carefully choosing occupations that are viewed as healthy and advantageous in child development (Millei & Lee, 2007). Occupational scientists could also take on this perspective to focus on risk at a global level; for example, investigating how some work occupations, associated with high environmental or health risks, become shifted from Western countries to countries with less complex, stringent or costly risk-management legislation.

In considering the potential contributions of the risk society perspective to the study of occupation, it is again important to consider its boundaries (Alexander, 1996; Lupton, 1999a). One relevant critique is that in neglecting cultural diversity, Beck assumed universalizing tendencies of a value consensus in risk society (Denney, 2005; Tulloch & Lupton, 2003). A second key critique highlights a lack of detail in historical analysis of how and why macro-level societal transformations have occurred. It is argued that Beck's lack of historical grounding misses other aspects of the social world, since it regards current risk consciousness as an inevitable result of an historical logic (Denney, 2005; O'Malley, 2000; Zinn, 2008). Both of these critiques point to the next two perspectives on risk; a cultural/symbolic perspective that forefronts risk as a cultural and collective concept, and a governmentality perspective that addresses risk as a technique of governing linked to power.

Cultural/symbolic perspective

Mary Douglas (1985, 1990, 1992; Douglas & Wildavsky, 1982), taking a cultural/symbolic perspective on risk, drew attention to risks as collective phenomena that are socially selected and constructed. She argued that concerns about risk are a result of cultural processes, and this makes it impossible to analyse risks without taking the uniqueness and values of the community in which the risks are perceived into account

(Denney, 2005). Rejecting a technico-scientific risk perspective, but stressing the social, cultural and political dimensions of risk, Douglas stated that risk is 'not only the probability of an event but also the probable magnitude of its outcome, and everything depends on the value that is set on the outcome' (Douglas, 1990, p. 10). Thus, taking a cultural/symbolic perspective on risk, it can be seen as 'a social process ... social principles that guide behavior affect the judgment of what dangers should be most feared, what risks are worth taking, and who should be allowed to take them' (Douglas & Wildavsky, 1982, p. 6).

Consequently, risk is viewed not as independent from but essentially *about* values, morals and politics. Douglas, highlighting social influences that select particular risks for attention, attempted to explain why some dangers are identified as 'risks', while others are not. She proposed that risk is a modern strategy to deal with danger and otherness that serves to construct and maintain boundaries between individual and social bodies (Lupton, 1999a). Referring to risk allows social groups, organizations and societies to deal with social deviance, to maintain their boundaries and achieve social order. As a powerful resource within normalization processes, risk can be understood as a modern blaming system. 'Under the new banner of risk reduction, a new blaming system has replaced the former combination of moralistic condemning the victim, and opportunistic condemning the victim's incompetence' (Douglas, 1992, p. 16).

In emphasizing the cultural context of risks, Douglas rejected models of risk that explain individual behaviour as determined by rational choice. Rather, Douglas argued that engaging in activities labelled as 'risky' by science and experts is not 'a weakness of understanding. It is a preference' (Douglas, 1985, p. 103). Taking cultural values and belief systems into consideration, decisions regarding risk cannot be considered as 'irrational' (Vahabi & Gastaldo, 2003). For example, an adolescent taking up the occupation of smoking might be well informed and aware of associated risks, but still engage in this occupation because of social meanings attached to smoking in particular cultures.

A cultural/symbolic perspective on risk highlights how different world views, mediated through value and belief systems and forms of social organization, generate different risk cultures. From this perspective, differences in risk assessment and risk acceptance between experts and lay people are not based on lacking or varying knowledge, but on fundamental 'culture-clashes' (Lupton, 1999a). Since risk represents collective belief systems, relative to culture and social position (Rosa, 1998), knowledge about risk is viewed as a social product, situated in a circumscribed social context.

Occupational scientists might find cultural/symbolic perspectives on risk valuable in studying how risk and occupation relate within socio-cultural processes. For example, they might research how occupation, when it is attached to risk, can carry out moral functions that maintain and convey a group's dominant values, such as health or responsibility. Drawing on the idea of risk as a strategy for normalization, scholars might research how risk is employed to 'other' or blame people who pursue occupations different to the dominant group within a given culture. For example, scholars might focus on how individuals who prefer 'deviant' occupations, such as tagging (Russell, 2008), become framed to be 'at'-risk for crime or addiction, and as 'a' risk to others. Occupational scientists could also study how social notions of risk shape the meaning of occupation for individuals in limiting, as well as enabling ways.

While a cultural/symbolic perspective on risk enables occupational scientists to move beyond a sole focus on individuals to consider risk as a socio-cultural concept, it has been critiqued for an over-emphasis on culture and for subsequently not attending adequately to the impact of social structures and personal traits on risk definitions and responses (Denney, 2005; Tulloch, 2008). The governmentality perspective on risk takes the critique of neglecting the hidden relationships between power, social position and collective claims on risk further, in that it focuses on risk as a technique to govern the conduct of individuals and groups.

Governmentality perspective

Governmentality theorists draw on Michel Foucault's analysis of how government of others and the self occurs (Lemke, 2002). Extending the idea of government significantly, Foucault viewed government as encompassing all modes of action that aim to shape, guide or direct the conduct of others and one's own towards certain ends (Foucault, 1991). Though Foucault did not explicitly address risk (Castel, 1991), authors have illustrated the usefulness of his analysis of governmentality in understanding the contemporary occurrence and permeation of risk in Western society. Different to the risk society perspective, which proposes that the increased preoccupation with risk is an effect of modernization, governmentality theorists argue that this increase reflects the rise of a particular mode of governing (Rothstein, Huber, & Gaskell, 2006). Risk is conceptualized as a calculative rationality; that is, as an organizing system of thought, rendering reality for particular ends to govern and 'colonize' the future (Ewald, 1991; Rothstein *et al.*, 2006). In turn, social authorities govern the conduct and subjectivities of individuals and collectives by prompting them to consider the risk of their actions and activities, so that they operate as rational, calculative and responsible citizens (Dannefer, 2000). Emphasizing the notion of risk as a rationality that shapes a particular reality for particular purposes, risk can be seen as:

> *a way, or rather, a set of different ways, of ordering reality, of rendering it into a calculable form. It is a way of representing events in a certain form so they might be made governable in particular ways, with particular techniques and for particular goals. It is a component of diverse forms of calculative rationality for governing the conduct of individuals, collectives and populations.* (Dean, 2010, p. 206)

The concept of discourse is central to the governmentality perspective. Discourses can be seen as identifiable ways of giving a particular meaning to reality through languages, ideas and images, based within a bounded body of knowledge, tied to particular political rationalities and associated social practices (Fairclough, 2001; Rose, 1999). Many authors point out that there has been an increasing use of risk in popular and expert discourses (Ericson & Haggerty, 1997; Garland, 2003; Skolbekken, 1995). As a type of discourse, discourses on risk operate as technologies of government that delimit and make possible what can be said and done about a phenomenon, and how people understand and govern themselves in relation to it. Thus, from a governmentality perspective, risk is seen as both a rationality and technology that produces and maintains power relations, particular types of subjectivities, conduct, and government of the self and others. Risk is seen as intimately connected to power; it facilitates patterns of self and other regulation that (re)produce power relations, and is enacted through a range of technologies, such as self-assessment, risk screening, or diagnostic processes that identify people as 'at risk'.

Like risk society theorists who point to the increasing individualization of risks in late modernity, governmentality theorists draw attention to the importance of the role of risk in promoting self-management. Yet governmentality theorists, such as Dean (1997) and O'Malley (1992), have linked the shift from socialized risk management to an increasing self-responsibility for avoiding and managing risks, to the political rationality of neoliberalism. Neoliberal approaches to government highlight a recession of the welfare state and promote minimal intervention on the part of the state by emphasizing individual responsibility, autonomy and self-reliance (Laliberte Rudman, 2005; Lupton, 1999a). Neoliberal rationality emphasizes individual responsibility to take control and prevent risk, within an ever increasing array of domains of life. As normalization is a central aspect of liberal government (Lupton, 1999b), those whose behaviour and choices deviate significantly from the norm will be identified as 'at risk'. Thus risk knowledge, provided by experts, becomes a technology of power, as it defines the boundaries of what is 'normal' and 'responsible' behaviour and what is 'risky' and 'irresponsible'.

Occupational scientists taking a governmentality perspective on risk might study how discourses about risk operate in the construction of subjectivity and social life through occupation. Forefronting risk as a powerful rationality that produces and maintains power relations could lead to critical interrogation of who benefits from encouraging individuals to make particular 'responsible' occupational choices. Or they might study how risk is employed in governing specific occupations of populations that are problematized as being 'at-risk' (such as driving in the elderly, or physical activity in children at risk for obesity). By focusing on occupations that have recently become problematized within risk discourses, scholars in occupational science could also research how risks and occupations come to be constructed differently in varying political contexts or across historical times.

One of the criticisms of a governmentality perspective on risk has been the tendency to focus on 'the blueprints for governments' (e.g., governmental policies or legislation) rather than 'descending' to see how people respond to discourses as part of their everyday lives (Denney, 2005; O'Malley, Weir, & Clifford, 1997). Another line of criticism argues that governmentality work tends not to attend to how differences in relation to gender, age, ethnicity interplay with how discourses are interpreted, presented, responded to or resisted (Lupton, 1999a).

Expanding ways of linking risk and occupation

We have demarcated four epistemological foundations of risk, bringing to light the key assumptions that inform research and action differently and considering the implications for the study of risk and occupation. Indeed, when occupational scientists link risk to occupation, it can make:

> *quite a difference whether we interpret risk as a result of new and recent types of risks we have to face, as a change in style of governance, as caused by an increasingly differentiated society, as a response of alienating conditions of living, or as a problem of diverse cultural interpretations.* (Zinn, 2008, p. 2)

The difference that Zinn highlighted is crucial for occupational scientists to reflect on when reading and engaging in work addressing risk, and underpins our assertion that ongoing discussion about each risk epistemology's contribution to the study of occupation is warranted.

As disciplinary mono-cultures can stifle knowledge generation, silence important voices and reproduce inequalities (Hammell, 2011; Laliberte Rudman *et al.*, 2008; Shiva, 1993), epistemological diversity is fundamental for the continued development of occupational science, as well as for its potential to address contemporary health and social concerns. Currently, a technico-scientific perspective on risk dominates many disciplinary discourses, such as medicine, health promotion, or public health (Lupton, 1995). Not surprisingly, a technico-scientific understanding of risk also seems to be prevalent in the occupation-based literature. Drawing on a technico-scientific understanding of risk, many authors have made valuable contributions in identifying risk factors connected to specific, absent or imbalanced occupations. Others have re-framed health risks, such as falls in the elderly, from an occupational perspective (Woodland & Hobson, 2003). While not negating the contributions of such work, it is also important to notice that alternative perspectives on risk are rare in works addressing risk and occupation (see, for example, Ballinger & Payne, 2000). While we argue for epistemological diversity when linking risk and occupation, we also believe that it is necessary to strengthen the use of critically oriented epistemologies to actively respond to current social concerns and the various ways risk is drawn upon to shape individual and collective occupations. As reviewed within this chapter, all three socio-cultural perspectives on risk provide a means to question the apparent neutrality of risk, and can be categorized as critically oriented.

Drawing upon critically oriented epistemologies on risk can create opportunities for new ways of thinking about and addressing risk within occupational science; ways that open up spaces for inclusion, equity and diversity – within and through occupation. To provide an example, all three critically oriented perspectives presented in this chapter raise awareness of how the identification of 'at-risk' individuals can, perhaps inadvertently, support individualization and 'victim-blaming' and contribute to the structural inequalities that shape individuals' vulnerability in the first place. Labelling individuals 'at-risk' within and through research can lead to locating 'problems', 'failures' or 'pathologies' related to occupations in individuals, families and communities rather than in institutional structures that create and maintain social and occupational inequalities. Further, the uncritical use of an at-risk label can foster marginalization as it often connotes an implicit need to save 'us' (the dominant group) from 'them' (the at-risk or risky other) by providing 'our' intervention and services (Lupton, 1999a).

Such tendencies, cultivated by a dominant technico-scientific perspective on risk, can be noticed in the occupation-based literature. For example, journal articles imply that 'we' need to be saved from the increasing health care costs 'they' produce by falling ('at-risk older adults', e.g. Clemson, Manor, & Fitzgerald, 2003); the accidents 'they' produce by still driving ('older drivers at risk for traffic violations', e.g. Lee & Lee, 2005); the unsafe neighbourhoods 'they' create by dropping out of school and engaging in harmful occupations ('at-risk youth', e.g. Snyder *et al.*, 1998); or the societal burden 'they' will become to 'us' by developing chronic diseases, due to 'their' physical inactivity or to 'their' parents' failure to raise adequately active children ('at-risk children', e.g. Poulsen & Ziviani, 2004). While all such articles are well intentioned in their aim to facilitate positive change *for* (or better: *in*) 'at-risk individuals' and their occupational repertoires, scholars outside occupational science have demonstrated how a generalized, sole and technico-scientific use of the at-risk label is highly problematic. For example, the label has been critiqued as 'implicitly racist, classist, sexist, and ableist' (Swadener & Lubeck, 1995, p. 3), as it frames the at-risk subject as universal and aims for normalization. As occupational scientists, we need to engage in a discussion of *whom* we conceptualize – and thus construct – in occupational science as being at-risk, on what basis such constructions are made, and what the implications of these constructions are for occupation. Reflecting on our current knowledge generation in occupational science, *why* do we think of particular individuals or social groups as being at-risk, and *what* exactly are they at-risk for?

Conclusion

In conclusion, the use of critically oriented epistemologies to inform the study of risk and occupation is particularly important within current societal transformations. Many authors propose that risk discourse is a 'seismic field' of society, raising concerns regarding how current risk discourses relate to and indicate fundamental social changes (Baker & Simon, 2002; Denney, 2005; Harthorn & Oaks, 2003). Denny (2005), for example, pointed out that concerns about the unsafe society have displaced concerns about equality in contemporary Western societies, and Baker and Simon (2002) called attention to the increasing variety of efforts to conceive and address social problems in terms of risk and make people individually accountable for risks.

Critical scholars, such as Rose (1996), have raised awareness of how dominant risk conceptualizations contribute to, and are reflexive of, neoliberal rationalities that promote an 'individualization of the social' related to re-configurations of welfare systems in many Western countries. Additionally, Peterson and Lupton (1996) have noted an increased visibility and influence of health promotion activities, critiquing their underlying moral and ideological content that shapes 'risky behaviour' as a failure to take care of the self. Others emphasize that the strong focus on individual lifestyles as a means to manage risk within the 'new public health' gives rise to individualism, behaviourism, consumerism and victim-blaming (Lupton, 1995; Petersen, 1997). Critically oriented perspectives on risk provide a valuable response to current societal challenges, as they facilitate occupational scientists to attend to macro-level contexts of occupation, such as modernization, culture and governance, and attend to the re-production of power relations in knowledge generation.

Acknowledgement

The first author would like to thank the members of her comprehensive exam advisory committee, Dr Jessica Polzer, Dr Thelma Sumsion and Dr Debbie Laliberte Rudman for their support of her doctoral work.

References

Adam, B., Beck, U., & Van Loon, J. (Eds). (2000). *The Risk Society and Beyond: Critical Issues for Social Theory*. London: Sage.

Alexander, J.C. (1996). Critical reflections on 'reflexive modernization'. *Theory Culture Society*, **13**, 133–8.

Baker, T., & Simon, J. (Eds). (2002). *Embracing Risk: The Changing Culture of Insurance and Responsibility*. Chicago: University of Chicago Press.

Ballinger, C., & Payne, S. (2000). Falling from grace or into expert hands? Alternative accounts about falling in older people. *British Journal of Occupational Therapy*, **63**, 573–9.

Beck-Gernsheim, E. (1996). Life as a planning project. In S. Lash, B. Szerszynski & B. Wynne (Eds), *Risk, Environment and Modernity: Towards a New Ecology* (pp. 139–53). Thousand Oaks, CA: Sage.

Beck, U. (1992). *Risk Society: Towards a New Modernity*. London: Sage.

Beck, U. (1999). *World Risk Society*. Cambridge: Polity Press.

Beck, U. (2002). The terrorist threat: World risk society revisited. *Theory Culture Society*, **19**, 39–55.

Bradbury, J.A. (1989). The policy implications of differing concepts of risk. *Science Technology Human Values*, **14**, 380–99.

Castel, R. (1991). From dangerousness to risk. In G. Burchell, C. Gordon & P. Miller (Eds), *The Foucault Effect: Studies in Governmentality* (pp. 281–98). Chicago: University of Chicago Press.

Clemson, L., Manor, D., & Fitzgerald, M.H. (2003). Behavioral factors contributing to older adults falling in public places. *OTJR Occupation, Participation and Health*, **23**, 107–17.

Dannefer, D. (2000). Bringing risk back in: The regulation of the self in the postmodern state. In K. Warner Schaie & J. Hendricks (Eds), *The Evolution of the Aging Self: The Societal Impact of the Aging Process* (pp. 269–80). New York: Springer.

Davis, R.M., & Pless, B. (2001). BMJ bans "accidents": Accidents are not unpredictable. *British Medical Journal*, **322**, 1320–1.

Dean, M. (1997). Sociology after society. In D. Owen (Ed.), *Sociology after Postmodernism* (pp. 205–28). Thousand Oaks, CA: Sage.

Dean, M. (2010). *Governmentality: Power and Rule in Modern Society* (2nd rev. ed.). Thousand Oaks, CA: Sage.

Denney, D. (2005). *Risk and Society*. Thousand Oaks, CA: Sage.

Douglas, M. (1985). *Risk Acceptability According to the Social Sciences*. London: Routledge & Kegan Paul.

Douglas, M. (1990). Risk as a forensic resource. *Daedalus*, **119**, 1–16.
Douglas, M. (1992). *Risk and Blame: Essays in Cultural Theory*. London: Routledge.
Douglas, M., & Wildavsky, A. (1982). *Risk and Culture: An Essay on the Selection of Technical and Environmental Dangers*. Berkeley: University of California Press.
Ericson, R.V., & Haggerty, K.D. (1997). *Policing the Risk Society*. Toronto: University of Toronto Press.
Ewald, F. (1991). Insurance and risk. In G. Burchell, C. Gordon & P. Miller (Eds), *The Foucault Effect: Studies in Governmentality* (pp. 197–210). Chicago: University of Chicago Press.
Fairclough, N. (2001). *Language and Power*. New York: Longman.
Foucault, M. (1991). Governmentality. In G. Burchell, C. Gordon & P. Miller (Eds), *The Foucault Effect: Studies in Governmentality* (pp. 87–104). Chicago: University of Chicago Press.
Furedi, F. (2002). *Culture of Fear: Risk-taking and the Morality of Low Expectation*. New York: Continuum.
Garland, D. (2003). The rise of risk. In R.V. Ericson & A. Doyle (Eds), *Risk and Morality* (pp. 48–86). Toronto: University of Toronto Press.
Giddens, A. (1990). *The Consequences of Modernity*. Stanford, CA: Stanford University Press.
Giddens, A. (1991). *Modernity and Self-identity: Self and Society in the Late Modern Age*. Cambridge, UK: Polity Press.
Gill, T. (2007). *No Fear: Growing Up in a Risk Averse Society*. London: Calouste Gulbenkian Foundation (UK Branch).
Hammell, K.W. (2011). Resisting theoretical imperialism in the disciplines of occupational science and occupational therapy. *British Journal of Occupational Therapy*, **74**, 27–33.
Harthorn, B.H., & Oaks, L. (2003). *Risk, Culture, and Health Inequality: Shifting Perceptions of Danger and Blame*. Westport, CN: Praeger.
Hilgartner, S. (1985). The political language of risk: Defining occupational health. In D. Nelkin (Ed.), *The Language of Risk* (pp. 25–65). Beverly Hills: Sage.
Jaeger, C. (2001). *Risk, Uncertainty, and Rational Action*. London: Earthscan.
Kellogg's Smart Start®. (2011). *Kellogg's Smart Start® Strong Heart Antioxidants cereal*. Retrieved 4 March 2011, from http://www2.kelloggs.com/Brand/brand.aspx?brand=212
Laliberte Rudman, D. (2005). Understanding political influences on occupational possibilities: An analysis of newspaper constructions of retirement. *Journal of Occupational Science*, **12**, 149–60.
Laliberte Rudman, D., Dennhardt, S., Fok, D. *et al.* (2008). A vision for occupational science: Reflecting on our disciplinary culture. *Journal of Occupational Science*, **15**, 136–46.
Lee, H.C., & Lee, A.H. (2005). Identifying older drivers at risk of traffic violations by using a driving simulator: A 3-year longitudinal study. *American Journal of Occupational Therapy*, **59**, 97–100.
Lemke, T. (2002). Foucault, governmentality, and critique. *Rethinking Marxism*, **14**, 49–64.
Levin, L. (2005). Life is a mixture of risks, what would a risk-free life be like? *Journal of Epidemiology and Community Health*, **59**, 1103.

Lupton, D. (1995). *The Imperative of Health: Public Health and the Regulated Body.* Thousand Oaks, CA: Sage.
Lupton, D. (1999a). *Risk.* London: Routledge.
Lupton, D. (Ed.). (1999b). *Risk and Sociocultural Theory: New Directions and Perspectives.* Cambridge: Cambridge University Press.
Millei, Z., & Lee, L. (2007). 'Smarten up the parents': Whose agendas are we serving? Governing parents and children through the Smart Population Foundation Initiative in Australia. *Contemporary Issues in Early Childhood*, 8, 208–21.
O'Brien, J., & Smith, J. (2002). Childhood transformed? Risk perceptions and the decline of free play. *British Journal of Occupational Therapy*, **65**, 123–8.
O'Byrne, P., & Holmes, D. (2007). The micro-fascism of Plato's good citizen: Producing (dis)order through the construction of risk. *Nursing Philosophy*, **8**, 92–101.
O'Malley, P. (1992). Risk, power and crime prevention. *Economy and Society*, **21**, 252–75.
O'Malley, P. (2000). Risk societies and the government of crime. In M. Brown & J. Pratt (Eds), *Dangerous Offenders: Punishment and Social Order* (pp. 17–34). London: Routledge.
O'Malley, P., Weir, L., & Clifford, S. (1997). Governmentality, criticism, policics. *Economy and Society*, **26**, 501–17.
Petersen, A. (1997). Risk, governance and the new public health. In A. Petersen & R. Bunton (Eds), *Foucault, Health and Medicine* (pp. 189–206). London: Routledge.
Petersen, A., & Lupton, D. (1996). *The New Public Health: Health and Self in the Age of Risk.* Thousand Oaks, CA: Sage.
Poulsen, A.A., & Ziviani, J.M. (2004). Health enhancing physical activity: Factors influencing engagement patterns in children. *Australian Occupational Therapy Journal*, **51**, 69–79.
Praeventia Bars. (2011). *Praeventia: A Taste of Life.* Retrieved 5 March 2011, from http://www.praeventia.ca
President's Choice On Track Cereal. (2011). *PC On Track Cereal.* Retrieved 5 March 2011, from http://www.presidentschoice.ca
Renn, O. (1992). Concepts of risk: A classification. In S. Krimsky & D. Golding (Eds), *Social Theories of Risk* (pp. 53–79). Westport, CT: Praeger.
Rosa, E.A. (1998). Metatheoretical foundations for post-normal risk. *Journal of Risk Research*, **1**, 15–44.
Rose, N. (1996). The death of the social? Re-figuring the territory of government. *Economy and Society*, **25**, 327–56.
Rose, N. (1999). *Powers of Freedom: Reframing Political Thought.* Cambridge: Cambridge University Press.
Rothstein, H., Huber, M., & Gaskell, G. (2006). A theory of risk colonization: The spiralling regulatory logics of societal and institutional risk. *Economy and Society*, **35**, 91–112.
Russell, E. (2008). Writing on the wall: The form, function and meaning of tagging. *Journal of Occupational Science*, **15**, 87–97.
Shiva, V. (1993). *Monocultures of the Mind: Perspectives on Biodiversity and Biotechnology.* London: Zed Books.

Skolbekken, J.-A. (1995). The risk epidemic in medical journals. *Social Science & Medicine*, **40**, 291–301.

Slovic, P. (1999). Trust, emotion, sex, politics, and science: Surveying the risk-assessment battlefield. *Risk Analysis*, **19**, 689–701.

Snyder, C., Clark, F., Masunaka-Noriega, M., & Young, B. (1998). Los Angeles street kids: New occupations for life program. *Journal of Occupational Science*, **5**, 133–9.

Swadener, B.B., & Lubeck, S. (Eds). (1995). *Children and Families "at promise": Deconstructing the Discourse of Risk*. New York: State University of New York Press.

Tulloch, J. (2008). Culture and risk. In J.O. Zinn (Ed.), *Social Theories of Risk and Uncertainty: An Introduction* (pp. 138–167). Oxford: Blackwell Publishing.

Tulloch, J., & Lupton, D. (2003). *Risk and Everyday Life*. Thousand Oaks, CA: Sage.

Vahabi, M., & Gastaldo, D. (2003). Rational choice(s)? Rethinking decision-making on breast cancer risk and screening mammography. *Nursing Inquiry*, **10**, 245–56.

Woodland, J.E., & Hobson, S.J.G. (2003). An occupational therapy perspective on falls prevention among community-dwelling older adults. *Canadian Journal of Occupational Therapy*, **70**, 174–82.

Workplace Safety & Insurance Board Ontario. (2008). *Road to Zero: A Prevention Strategy for Workplace Health and Safety in Ontario 2008–2012*. Retrieved 4 March 2011, from http://www.wsib.on.ca

Zinn, J.O. (Ed.). (2008). *Social Theories of Risk and Uncertainty: An Introduction*. Oxford: Blackwell Publishing.

Part IV

Ways of doing in occupational science

10 The case for multiple research methodologies

Valerie A. Wright-St Clair

Listening to the philosophical meanings within Leunig's (2001) letter from the imaginary Mr Curly of Curly Flat to his friend, Vasco Pyjama, provides a good starting point for considering the case for multiple methodologies in occupational science. The letter begins:

> *Dear Vasco, it is the shortest day here in Curly Flat – the winter solstice. We had a very interesting time trying to measure the shortest day. How does one measure a day? Length is one matter but depth and width are just as important. For instance, a short day may be very deep or a long day may be shallow and narrow. What seems to be vital is whether or not the day is spacious, in which case the roundedness of the day is perhaps the most important factor.* (Leunig, 2001, p. 49)

Leunig's whimsical letter points toward important phenomena and questions for occupational scientists to grapple with. Some come to mind. What is one measuring when setting out to understand occupation and how ought things be measured? How can we come to know something of the 'length' of occupation, or of its 'depth' or 'breadth' for that matter? Could it be that what is measured merely proffers a shallow and narrow knowledge of occupation? And, how might we come to know occupation in its fullness or 'roundedness'? The quality of roundedness indicates an understanding of occupation that encapsulates knowledge of length and depth and breadth all together. Each dimensional perspective

Occupational Science: Society, Inclusion, Participation, First Edition.
Edited by Gail Whiteford and Clare Hocking.

reveals something the others do not. Roundedness suggests both the stillness of coming to 'know' occupation in itself, and the restlessness of seeking to know occupation in ways that are not yet understood. Roundedness symbolizes, paradoxically, qualities of being encapsulated within a boundary yet, at the same time, being spacious and open to expansion or contraction. And, as with the hermeneutic circle (Gadamer, 1975/2004), coming to understand the parts of knowledge about occupation suggests a greater understanding of the whole of it will be gained; while grasping some of its wholeness will lend different and deeper ways to understand the parts.

This chapter begins by exploring the meaning of occupational science being a 'science' and how different research questions can serve the development of occupational science knowledge. The complexity of identifying what is and what is not occupational science research is discussed. Then, in making the case for multiple methodologies, a forward-looking framework for occupational science's research agenda is used to illustrate how one core question, the relationship between occupation and health, might be examined and potentially explained. Rather than occupational science knowledge growing organically, as has predominantly occurred, the way forward will be best served by the considered exploration of socially relevant questions, which calls for the use of multiple research methodologies.

The science in occupational science

Before moving on to consider the case for multiple methodologies, it is worth stepping back to think about what it means for occupational science to be a 'science.' Stemming from the Latin word *scientia*, science means 'knowledge' (Onions, 1966, p. 797). Therefore occupational science, as a science, is concerned with the methodical processes related to building knowledge. The inclusion of science in the name indicates the field holds itself up to be involved in the scientific endeavour. At its most simplistic, the scientific endeavour is the pursuit of understanding, explaining and predicting things in the world (Okasha, 2002). From a conventional, empiricist viewpoint, the scientific nature of occupational science would mean it was underpinned by the fundamental assumption that objective realities or truths about human occupation exist. Accordingly, the research methods used would be characterized by objectivity, and analysing observational data received through the senses, 'independent of thinking and thoughts' (Hung, 2006, p. 3). While this perspective is widely adhered to in Western societies, it fails to encapsulate contemporary understandings of what it is that makes occupational science, or other sciences, scientific by nature.

Two decades ago, the American Association for the Advancement of Science (AAAS) (as cited in Gauch, 2003) espoused a more liberal view by defining science as 'the art of interrogating nature' (p. 98). From this standpoint, occupational science would be characterized by questioning, but not just any questioning; thoughtful, methodical questioning of things within the field of interest. This fundamentally different viewpoint means science is more than the production of knowledge by way of a rigorous sequence of research steps. It reframes science as a liberal 'art' (Gauch, 2003). In accord with this idea, occupational science, like other sciences, would be a 'highly creative endeavour' (AAAS, 1993/2009). Multiple and highly variable pathways would be open to occupational scientists engaging in the process of knowledge production. Phenomena of interest would be 'multiply realizable' (Hitchcock, 2004, p. 160), and hence, open to a multiplicity of research methodologies arising from different types of questions. From this liberal viewpoint, scientists doing occupational science would differ:

> *in how they go about their work; in the reliance they place on historical data or on experimental findings and on qualitative or quantitative methods; in their recourse to fundamental principles; and in how much they draw on the findings of other sciences* ... [yet there would be] *common understandings among them about what constitutes an investigation that is scientifically [trustworthy].* (AAAS, 1989/1990a, cited in Hitchcock, 2004, p. 160)

Thinking of science as the art of questioning or interrogating things in the world also suggests that occupational science's scientific endeavour is more than the research itself. Questions do not just appear out of nowhere; they arise from particular interests which in turn are embedded in historical and philosophical contexts (Gauch, 2003). In other words, it can be assumed that all science is underpinned by conceptual ideas and theoretical frameworks which reveal and restrict the field of interest. Therefore, doing occupational science would also involve developing and articulating theory, conducting thought experiments (Hitchcock, 2004) related to the application of theory, and the thoughtful derivation of new phenomena of interest (Hung, 2006). The theoretical and the methodological cannot be disentangled in the quest for understanding things in the world. Furthermore, common sense suggests not all things in the world are observable. As a consequence, the case is strengthened for raising different types of questions which call for the creative, considered use of multiple methodologies.

Naming occupational science, as a science, is a hopeful standpoint. It shows a confidence that there are innumerable things to be explored within the field of interest. It expresses an assumption that things of interest in the world can be, at least partially, known and understood. And it lays the foundation for building a research methodology repertoire that is at once diverse and seemingly limitless in subtleties of design.

The occupation in occupational science

Until now, the discussion has focused on what makes occupational science a science. The next question seems to be what is it that makes this science occupational in nature? To be a field of interest, something must act to bring the otherwise disparate science activities into connection and to bind things together. The notion that all science is carried out within a 'paradigm,' or overarching theoretical framework, seems to help (Hung, 2006). First described by Kuhn (as cited in Gauch, 2003), a paradigm is 'a strong network of commitments – conceptual, theoretical, instrumental, and methodological' (p. 84). So what is it that occupational scientists collectively hold an allegiance to? What forms the common ground and unites occupational science in its scientific endeavour? Clark (2006) asserted that 'occupation' is occupational science's 'unifying operative paradigm' (p. 170). Looking at the occupational science literature suggests a 'strong network of commitments' does exist. While the topics are highly variable, the theoretical discussions and research questions circle around explorations and explanations of human occupation. The fact that there is not one, universally accepted, definition of 'occupation' could be seen to destabilize the scientific foundations.

However, the view I would put forward is that multiple, sometimes competing, definitions serve the scientific endeavour. Occupational science may only flourish in a context in which divergent views are voiced and debated and knowledge development is celebrated as being continually in flux. Rather than trying to seek certainties, occupational science will be best served by theorists and researchers who embrace scientific uncertainty, accept all knowledge is merely an approximation of things which are multiply realizable, and make a commitment to the continual revision of knowledge (AAAS, 1989/1990a; Gauch, 2003). While occupational scientists ought to reject the idea of finding and explaining absolute truths (AAAS, 1989/1990a), it is significant that some 'truths' endure. For example, the presupposition that humans are essentially occupational beings (Molineux & Whiteford, 2011; Yerxa *et al.*, 1989) binds the thinking and doing of occupational science.

As well as 'knowledge,' science may have originally meant 'to separate one thing from another, to distinguish' (Harper, 2010). In this way, occupational science ought to be distinguishable from other sciences. As a young science, it seems the boundaries of what is occupational science knowledge, and what is not, are yet to be collectively defined. Accepting, as the distinguishing characteristic, that occupational science 'is ultimately concerned with the exploration of human occupation in its totality' (Molke, Laliberte Rudman, & Polatajko, 2004, p. 277) suggests the field is bounded but not tightly constrained. Returning to the opening thoughts, holding such a distinction seems to encourage a rounded approach to the scientific endeavour, allowing the restlessness of exploration of occupation in ways that are not yet understood. Indeed, the parameters of occupation open to study are varied and still expanding (Hocking, 2009). As knowledge within occupational science develops it is important to leave the field open to ways of knowing the totality of occupation that are not yet visible. Nonetheless, unless the parts of research knowledge cluster together into a complex, unified whole, occupational science is at risk of losing its way as a distinguishable scientific field. The use of multiple methodologies alone might serve the development of knowledge, but it is not enough to bring about the roundedness of occupational science without human occupation as its distinguishing and unifying paradigm.

Occupational science activity

In everyday language, scientific activity is sometimes spoken of in terms of being 'hard' science or 'soft' science; the former referring to methods using deductive inquiry and the latter to forms of inductive, interpretive inquiry. Yet these colloquial expressions are unhelpful as they suggest one form is inherently more valuable than the other. Speaking of scientific activity as being hard science holds connotations of it being rigorous and durable, giving a solid knowledge foundation. On the other hand, saying science activity is soft science carries nuances of it being limp or flexible, yielding weak knowledge. The language of scientific activity needs to move beyond such value-laden distinctions.

Interestingly, a systematic comparison of named 'occupational science' articles published in the years 1990 and 2000, revealed, at each point in time, only 30% could be classified as reporting basic or, in a minority of cases, applied research activity (Molke *et al.*, 2004). This means over two-thirds of occupational science publications in both years, a decade apart, were discussion-based or theoretical in nature. In a similar systematic analysis of publications across the decade from 1996 to 2006, nearly 44% were classified as research (Glover, 2009). The findings of these two studies are not directly comparable as they used different approaches, so it cannot be concluded that occupational science research activity increased by 14% between 2000 and 2006. However, the second study did show a significant increase in the proportion of research articles published during the later period of 2003 to 2006 (Glover, 2009). But not all occupational science research makes it to publication. In an almost identical timeframe, 2002 to 2006, an analysis of the scholarly presentations at the annual Society for the Study of Occupation: USA (SSO:USA) symposia revealed 59% were research-based (Pierce *et al.*, 2010). While the trend looks promising, taken together, these analyses suggest occupational science's research-informed knowledge, as compared to its theory-based knowledge, is underdeveloped. This seeming imbalance may be a natural consequence of the emergent nature of the scientific field; the early thinking prepares the ground from which research questions grow.

Given the assumed complexity of human occupation, and thus the richness of understandings to be mined, occupational science has always stood on the ground of being an interdisciplinary academic discipline. Such an approach 'demands a fresh synthesis of interdisciplinary perspectives to provide a coherent corpus of knowledge about occupation' (Zemke & Clark, 1996, p. ix). The full potential of interdisciplinary research collaboration lies before occupational scientists and is still emphasized as holding the most promise in the way forward (Molke *et al.*, 2004). Working in partnership with scientists from different academic disciplines to 'interrogate' human occupation in its totality bodes well in the scientific endeavour of uncovering new questions to ask. Inevitably, a rich diversity of scientific questions will call for using a multiplicity of methodologies in order to best answer the questions raised. To illustrate, bringing an occupational science focus to the field of sport and recreation is leading to innovative work being done on understanding the consumer behaviour, or occupations, of sports fans (Humphries & Smith, 2006). Interpreting 'sport fandom' as an occupation offers a fresh way for event managers to take account of the meaning of what fans do.

The call for multiple methodologies

> *An enormous multiplicity of strands of evidence, many of them weak and ambiguous, can make a coherent logical bond whose strength is enormous.* (Gauch, 2003, p. 93)

The call for using multiple research methodologies within the emergent discipline of occupational science is nothing new (Clark, 2006; Glover, 2009; Wilcock, 2003; Zemke & Clark, 1996). From its inception, the place of 'qualitative' research methodologies was claimed to be 'more suited than experimental methods for the study of occupation because of occupation's richness in symbolic meanings' (Zemke & Clark, 1996, p. viii). This premise seems to live out in the nature of research produced in the name of occupational science. In a systematic quantitative analysis of the research, starting with the year of occupational science's inception, Molke *et al.* (2004) found 'in 1990 all three research articles were classified as quantitative, while in 2000 three were quantitative, two were mixed and eight were qualitative in nature' (p. 274). It is surprising that, in spite of the increase in research activity within the field, the number of 'quantitative' studies published remained the same a decade later. Similarly, Glover's (2009) analysis of the decade ending in 2006 found just over 70% of occupational science research publications employed a qualitative research methodology. The proportion is greater again in Pierce and colleagues' (2010) analysis of the first five years of SSO:USA meetings, where 84% were found to be qualitative in nature. This means only 1 in 13 scholarly presentations reported results of quantitative research. A further 1 in 10 used a mixed methods design. However, discussing occupational science research in terms of a quantitative–qualitative dichotomy is unhelpful for illuminating the multiplicity of methodologies being used. Usefully, Pierce *et al.*, throw a light on the qualitative methodologies underpinning the SSO:USA presentations. Grounded theory was most common, used in one out of five studies, followed by narrative inquiry, phenomenology and ethnography. Yet, going a step further, the call for merely using multiple methodologies is a hollow one in the absence of a greater purpose for doing occupational science research. So, what are occupational scientists called to question and why?

The call to question

The scope of what occupational science is called to question is pointed to within the International Society of Occupational Science's (Asaba *et al.*, 2007) definition of occupation as 'the various everyday activities people do as individuals, in families and within communities to occupy time and bring meaning and purpose to life' (p. 1). Inherent in the words are philosophical assumptions about occupational science's human, social and political responsibilities. For occupational science to be relevant within the societies it serves, the call to question occupation in its fullness is to identify the questions that matter for humanity. At the end of the day, 'a science that asks life's big questions is more human and more appealing than an impoverished science divorced from the humanities' (Gauch, 2003, p. 154). Judgements regarding occupational science's human, social and political relevance will rest with its potential to address, at least in part, the big challenges faced by humans and nations.

So what are some of the pressing global and local challenges facing human kind? The list is expansive and disquieting. Many challenges relate to reducing the threats toward international peace and security such as eradicating the global growth of organized crime and drug trafficking, terrorism, and civil conflict (UN, 2010). Others are concerned with promoting fundamental human rights such as protecting the cultural rights of indigenous peoples, the humane treatment of asylum seekers and refugees, the protection of children affected by poverty and conflict, the equality of women's social participation, the protection against sexual abuse and exploitation, the elimination of human trafficking (UN, 2010), and the reduction of HIV-related stigma and discrimination (UNESCO, 2010). Yet other challenges relate to global ecology such as responding responsibly to climate change, natural resource degradation, population growth and the changing age structure of populations, human displacement and homelessness following natural disasters, and the increasing urbanization of populations (Worldwatch Institute, 2008). Lastly, a further cluster of challenges relate to social development for improving the everyday lives of young people, families, older people, and people with disabilities, reducing youth unemployment, creating sustainable communities, eradicating poverty (UN, 2010), promoting basic literacy and education for all peoples, building community capacity (UNESCO, 2010), promoting equitable health development, and fostering water, food and health security (WHO, 2010).

Science, and by implication, occupational science, has its part to play in creating a better world for all. Looking forward, 'what the future holds in store for individual human beings, the nation, and the world depends largely on the wisdom with which humans use science and technology' (AAAS, 1989/1990b). In accord with this view, occupational scientists are already vocal in their concern for addressing occupationally focused, social justice issues; in other words, 'occupational justice'. Molineux and Whiteford's (2011) proposal for the occupational science research agenda to be guided by a framework consistent with 'the levels at which occupation occurs and is organized' (p. 247) means questions would be raised across a matrix of concerns facing individuals, families, communities and populations. Contemporary approaches to public health research suggest the levels of 'organizations' and 'policy' be added when studying a comprehensive array of health determinants and disparities (Steckler & Linnan, 2002). In fact, the sheer complexity and diversity of what ought to be explored within an occupational science research agenda (Molineux & Whiteford, 2011) means the full repertoire of methodologies will be called for in the scientific endeavour. The following section focuses on one overarching concern and, in doing so, illustrates how the case for multiple methodologies in occupational science is cemented.

Questioning the relationship between occupation and healthfulness

One enduring idea underpinning occupational science is the assumed relationship between the engagement in occupation and the healthfulness of peoples and populations (Wilcock, 1993; Yerxa, 1998). This essential claim demands a central place within occupational science's research agenda (Molineux & Whiteford, 2011). Bringing together some of the big challenges facing human kind, the levels at which occupation occurs, and the demand to understand the association between human occupation and healthfulness, reveals how multiple methodologies must be used to take occupational science forward in a socially relevant way.

The individual, occupation and health

In 2009, under the United Nations High Commissioner for Refugees (UNHCR) programme, 112 400 refugees were resettled across 19 nations (UNHCR Division of Programme Support & Management, 2010). The resettled individuals, one third of whom were Iraqi, highlight the plight of more than 10 million refugees living in, often prolonged, asylum (UNHCR Division of Programme Support & Management, 2010). Resettlement in a 'third country' is the last option. Each year, Australia, Canada, Finland, New Zealand, Norway, Sweden, the United Kingdom, the United States and other host States, participate in the global humanitarian effort by offering a new start in a new place. Occupationally, as the challenge of everyday living in refuge ends, that of making the host country 'home' is just beginning. Importantly, diverse research evidence suggests individuals' trauma recovery, health and well-being can be positively influenced by the resettlement experience (Sampson & Gifford, 2010). Yet resettlement is a slow, intricate process with a mix of State and Non-Governmental Organizations typically offering 'cultural orientation, language and vocational training as well as programmes to promote access to education and employment' (UNHCR: The UN Refugee Agency, 2010).

Occupational science is thriving in the major resettlement nations, and therefore is well placed to support this pressing humanitarian endeavour. Approaches that describe or address the subtleties of everyday living, social participation, individuals' traditional and new occupational needs and expectations, or the meaning of participation in otherwise hidden, everyday occupations have the potential to add value to existing resettlement efforts. Research methodologies such as ethnography, using in-depth individual, or focus group, interviews and participant observation to understand cultural phenomena such as how participation in everyday occupations influences ethnic identity for recently resettled refugees, or what influence cultural diversity has on occupational patterns within local communities, may reveal new occupationally focused understandings to inform resettlement programmes. On the other hand, epidemiological methodologies or secondary analysis of existing data might be used to build an understanding of the pattern and prevalence of refugee settlement in local communities. Survey methods such as such community mapping would give information about local amenities and environmental resources. Ultimately, other than building knowledge itself, descriptive occupational science research has the greater potential to inform applied studies and occupationally focused programmes aimed at advancing the healthfulness of people from refugee backgrounds.

The family, occupation and health

Research suggests that, for young people, sitting down with the family for meals and eating breakfast are associated with a better nutritional profile that continues into adulthood (Adolescent Health Research Group, 2008). From an occupational perspective this implies that food occupations within the home context are an important predictor of health and well-being outcomes. Recently, a large, representative survey-based study of New Zealand secondary school students revealed concerning results. 'Just over half the students reported that their family ate meals together on 5 or more days in the past week' (Adolescent Health Research Group, 2008, p. 19). Their food occupations were associated with social index. Compared with other students, those from more deprived neighbourhoods were twice as likely to buy their breakfast from takeaway bars or shops rather than eat at home.

Occupational science might contribute meaningfully to understanding and changing this social pattern of food occupations in a multiplicity of ways. Two are suggested. A grounded theory approach, gathering in-depth data from families across the social spectrum, could build an understanding of the processes involved in making decisions about meals and meal times. Working with this knowledge, an evidence-based occupational science (Clark, Jackson, & Carlson, 2004) study could be conducted to test the effectiveness of different family-focused, occupation-centred interventions aimed at making family meal times routine, daily events. Clark and her team at the University of Southern California articulated and continue to refine the strategies for occupational science evidence-based practice. They advocate using a strategic sequence of different methodologies including a comprehensive literature review, an exploratory interpretive study and a randomized controlled trial to test the efficacy of the carefully designed interventions. Follow-up surveys could be used to determine the ongoing outcomes and cost-effectiveness of the interventions.

The community, occupation and health

Increasingly, communities around the globe are home to culturally diverse peoples as a consequence of migration, refugee resettlement, family reunification and other reasons. Yet, while cultural diversity may advance the health of communities through economic, cultural and spiritual development (UNESCO, 2010), reports of exclusionary attitudes and practices in communities are prevalent (Boat People SOS, 2009). For example, in the United Kingdom, racially motivated incidents are played out on the streets of rural and urban communities (Athwal, Bourne, & Wood, 2010). Research of 660 cases reported during 2009 demonstrated they were typically 'random acts of unprovoked violence, carried out by mainly young white men' (Athwal *et al.*, 2010, p. 6) acting alone or in groups. The attacks varied in nature from 'graffiti on a wall and spoken abuse to the clandestine setting of fires and violent, murderous stabbings' (Athwal *et al.*, 2010, p. 10). Young adults and youth were also highly represented amongst the victims, particularly 'refugees, asylum seekers, migrant workers or overseas students' (Athwal *et al.*, 2010, p. 7). Internationally, disaffected young people, often in areas of high youth unemployment, contribute significantly to community instability (UN, 2010).

Thinking of 'victimizing' as an occupation suggests a place for occupational science in attempting to understand and resolve this widespread issue. One methodological approach would be to use phenomenology to understand the community-based experiences of those doing the victimizing and how the occupation fits within the everyday comings and goings of the local community. Such understandings could be used to develop occupationally focused interventions at a community level. However, a local need for inclusive forms of cultural diversity might be best served by truly collaborative, community-based participatory research (Minkler & Wallerstein, 2003). By way of the methodological interplay between research and action, the methods would be aimed at empowering the local community to collectively address young people's participation in victimizing occupations, and in building the community's capacity for creating health-promoting occupations for its own people.

The population, occupation and health

In almost all countries in the world, the proportion of people aged 60 and older is increasing. Older adults currently number over 700 million, or about 11% of the global population. By the middle of this century it is expected that this number will grow to 2 billion, meaning older adults will constitute 22% of all the world's peoples (UN DESA, 2009). Accordingly, promoting a healthful life for its older members is an important matter for most societies (UN Programme on Ageing, 2007). Much of the international research examines the biological, medical and social determinants of older adults' health. However, several large studies suggest participation in occupations may be an important determinant of healthfulness in advanced age (Glass *et al.*, 1999; Haggblom-Kronlof & Sonn, 2005; Menec, 2003).

One current longitudinal, cohort study of older New Zealanders, Maori aged 80–90 years and non-Maori turning 85, offers the hope of new insights into the relationship between occupation and health. Led by Ngaire Kerse at the University of Auckland, the researchers have recruited a sample of almost 1000 older adults living within several defined geographic boundaries. As an interdisciplinary project, the study aims to determine what the predictors of 'successful' advanced ageing are, and what the relative importance of health, social, occupational and environmental variables, and cultural practices are in predicting healthy ageing. Comprehensive, face-to-face interviews are being conducted in people's place of residence by local research assistants, trained to implement all the measures. Funding has been secured for gathering follow-up data at 12 months, in 2011, and again at 24 months. The plan is to follow the participants through to end of life. While the interplay of health, social, occupational, environmental and cultural variables in everyday life is complex, longitudinal, cohort methodologies hold the prospect of explaining the role of different occupations and occupational participation in promoting the healthfulness of populations.

Bringing the research conversation together

Good research is being done in the name of occupational science. There is more research within the field that is entirely congruent but not named as occupational science when it comes to publication. The naming is one step easily made in raising the prevalence and visibility of occupational science research. Occupational science growth over its first two decades is predominantly in research using interpretive approaches. While this emphasis does contribute to occupational science being distinguishable for its strengths in the interpretive paradigm, the pattern suggests a pressing need for opening up the range of questions being asked and, therefore, the diversity of research methodologies being used. Greater interdisciplinary collaboration in researching occupation may be one impetus for this to occur (Clark, 2006; Molke *et al.*, 2004). Other disciplines such as population health, human geography, gerontology and neuroscience have a history of raising particular types of questions and building strengths in research methodologies such as epidemiology, cross-sectional studies, prospective cohort studies, retrospective case control studies, randomized controlled trials and process evaluations.

The synthesis of knowledge generated from interdisciplinary research collaborations, as is already occurring, will continue to bring fresh ways of asking about occupation, new ways of researching it, and yield yet-to-be-discovered ways of implementing occupation-focused interventions at the level of the individual, the family, the community, and the population. For example, Clark (2006) made a case for policy-directed, strategic collaborations enabling '"big science" with real world applications' (p. 176). At the end of the day, it is the roundedness of the knowledge of occupation that matters. Keeping occupation as the concept that unifies occupational science research will avoid intellectual fragmentation (Clark, 2006).

Using the language of science is important. When looking at occupational science research publications underpinned by positivism the research designs are not named as being 'quantitative' in nature. In the positivist tradition the study designs are named; such as a pre-test–post-test survey (Frank *et al.*, 2008), a '2 x 2 repeated measures design' (Persch *et al.*, 2009, p. 163), an 'instrumental case study design' (Wood, Womack, & Hooper, 2009, p. 339), a 'prospective cohort study' (Glass *et al.*, 1999, p. 478), or a 'randomized controlled trial' (Clark *et al.*, 1997, p. S74). When the design is named, research methods that contribute to the trustworthiness of the study as a whole are known. Granted, positivism has a long history and the research designs typically align with long-established traditions, but it does mean the foundations for research rigour are rendered more visible and therefore more readily open to critique. The same needs to occur with occupational science research conducted within the interpretive paradigm. Rather than naming studies as being 'qualitative' in nature, the methodological approach ought to be named and clearly described, such as Glaserian grounded theory, or Foucauldian discourse analysis or Heiddegerian phenomenology; opening the methods up to rigorous application and review.

While this chapter has illustrated how diversifying the questions asked will necessarily lead to the use of a rich repertoire of research methodologies, the true value of embracing multiple methodologies will only be realized when the relevant philosophy or methodology is rigorously applied from beginning to end. The inception of occupational science as a science already implies the existence of 'trustworthy methods for the discovery of new truth within its own domain' (Simpson & Weiner, 1989, p. 649). It is time to more fully claim and demonstrate the 'science' in occupational science. The work has begun in earnest; however, there is a long way to go before occupational science is fully living up to its name.

Viewing occupation through the different methodological lenses available ought to be like looking through a kaleidoscope. With each methodological turn, different pieces of knowledge will fall into place, allowing some things to be seen and other things to be concealed. Like the pieces of coloured glass in the kaleidoscope, the methodological scope for knowing occupation in its roundedness, its entirety, is colourful and of endless variety. To build a robust science for the betterment of humanity, occupational scientists must continue to define the research agenda within local and global contexts, diversify the research questions being asked, and invest heavily in research excellence using the rich and creative array of possible research methodologies.

What seems important is the assumption that we can only ever be on the way to knowing human occupation in it wholeness. 'A complete understanding can never be fully realized, as human occupation is infinite in nature' (Molke *et al.*, 2004, p. 277). The task of occupational science, as a science, will never be done. While this may sound daunting, it is this 'always being on the way to understanding' nature that delivers occupational scientists over to the excitement of doing occupational science; of pondering deeply and of doing the research. And it is this yearning to grasp occupation, more and more fully in its wholeness, which opens up the possibilities for knowing it. It is the incessant journey towards understanding the roundedness of occupation, in yet-to-be-known ways, which matters to occupational science.

The ideas shared in this chapter are but one small part of an evolving, and necessary, critical conversation about occupational science. This thought brings the case for multiple methodologies back to the words of Leunig's (2001) Mr Curly:

> *Once again Vasco, it is not the length of life which is important, it is the shape and the spaciousness – for therein lies the potential for a beautiful freedom. It is the roundedness of life that matters. A round life is surely a happy life – and dare I say – it is a good life. Please consider these reflections as a small picnic of thoughts we may share together.* (p. 50)

References

Adolescent Health Research Group. (2008). *Youth'07: The Health and Wellbeing of Secondary School Students in New Zealand. Initial Findings.* Auckland: The University of Auckland.

American Association for the Advancement of Science (AAAS). (1989/1990a). *Science for all Americans Online. Chapter 1: The Nature of Science.* Retrieved from http://www.project2061.org/publications/sfaa/online/chap1.htm (last accessed 25 June 2011).

American Association for the Advancement of Science (AAAS). (1989/1990b). *Science for all Americans Online. Introduction.* Retrieved from http://www.project2061.org/publications/sfaa/online/intro.htm (last accessed 25 June 2011).

American Association for the Advancement of Science (AAAS). (1993/2009). *Benchmarks Online: Project 2061.* Retrieved from http://www.project2061.org/publications/bsl/online/index.php?chapter=1#B0 (last accessed 25 June 2011).

Asaba, E., Blanche, E., Jonsson, H., Laliberte Rudman, D., & Wicks, A. (2007). *The Way Forward Plan for ISOS, the International Society for Occupational Science.* Retrieved from http://isos.nfshost.com/Policy.html (last accessed 25 June 2011).

Athwal, H., Bourne, J., & Wood, R. (2010). *Racial Violence: The Buried Issue.* Retrieved from http://www.irr.org.uk/pdf2/IRR_Briefing_No.6.pdf (last accessed 25 June 2011).

Boat People SOS. (2009). *Boat People SOS Joins Community Protests against Racially Motivated Violence in Philadelphia*: BPSOS. Retrieved from http://www.bpsos.org/en/media-room/press-releases?start=10 (last accessed 25 June 2011).

Clark, F. (2006). One person's thoughts on the future of occupational science. *Journal of Occupational Science*, **13**, 167–79.

Clark, F., Azen, S.P., Zemke, R. *et al.* (1997). Occupational therapy for independent-living older adults: A randomised controlled trial. *Journal of the American Medical Association*, **278**, 1321–6.

Clark, F., Jackson, J., & Carlson, M. (2004). Occupational science, occupational therapy and evidence-based practice: What the well elderly study has taught us. In M. Molineux (Ed.), *Occupation for Occupational Therapists* (pp. 200–18). Oxford: Blackwell Publishing.

Frank, G., Murphy, S., Kitching, H.J., Garfield, D.M., & McDarment, N. (2008). The Tule River Tribal History Project: Evaluating a California Tribal Government's collaboration with anthropology and occupational therapy to preserve indigenous history and promote tribal goals. *Human Organization*, **67**, 430–42. doi:0018-7259/08/040430-13$1.80/1

Gadamer, H.-G.(1975/2004). *Truth and Method* (trans. J. Weinsheimer & D.G. Marshall). London: Continuum.

Gauch, H. G. (2003). *Scientific Method in Practice*. Cambridge: Cambridge University Press.

Glass, T.A., Mendes de Leon, C., Marottoli, R.A., & Berkman, L.F. (1999). Population-based study of social and productive activities as predictors of survival among elderly Americans. *British Medical Journal*, **319**, 478–83. doi:1999:319:478-83.

Glover, J.S. (2009). The literature of occupational science: A systematic, quantitative examination of peer-reviewed publications from 1996–2006. *Journal of Occupational Science*, **16**, 92–103.

Haggblom-Kronlof, G., & Sonn, U. (2005). Interests that occupy 86-year-old persons living at home: Associations with functional ability, self-rated health and sociodemographic characteristics. *Australian Occupational Therapy Journal*, **53**, 196–204. doi:10.1111/j.1440-1630.2005.00526.x

Harper, D. (Ed.). (2010). *Online Etymology Dictionary*. Retrieved from http://www.etymonline.com/index.php?search=science&searchmode=nl (last accessed 3 July 2011).

Hitchcock, C. (Ed.). (2004). *Contemporary Debates in Philosophy of Science*. Oxford: Blackwell Publishing.

Hocking, C. (2009). The challenge of occupation: Describing the things people do. *Journal of Occupational Science*, **16**, 140–50.

Humphries, C.E., & Smith, A.C.T. (2006). Sport fandom as an occupation: Understanding the sport consumer through the lens of occupational science. *International Journal of Sport Management and Marketing*, **1**, 331–48.

Hung, E.H.C. (2006). *Beyond Kuhn: Scientific Explanation, Theory Structure, Incommensurability and Physical Necessity*. Aldershot: Ashgate Publishing.

Leunig, M. (2001). *The Curly Pyjama Letters*. Ringwood, Australia: Viking.

Menec, V.H. (2003). The relation between everyday activities and successful aging: A 6-year longitudinal study. *The Journals of Gerontology*, **58B**, S74–S82.

Minkler, M., & Wallerstein, N. (2003). Introduction to community-based participatory research. In M. Minkler & N. Wallerstein (Eds), *Community-Based Participatory Research for Health* (pp. 3–26). San Francisco: Jossey-Bass.

Molineux, M., & Whiteford, G. (2011). Occupational science: Genesis, evolution and future contribution. In E. Duncan (Ed.), *Foundation for Practice in Occupational Therapy* (5th ed., pp. 243–253). Edinburgh: Churchill Livingstone.

Molke, D.K., Laliberte Rudman, D., & Polatajko, H. (2004). The promise of occupational science: A developmental assessment of an emerging academic discipline. *Canadian Journal of Occupational Therapy*, **71**, 269–81.

Okasha, S. (2002). *Philosophy of Science: A Very Short Introduction.* Oxford: Oxford University Press.

Onions, C.T. (Ed.). (1966). *The Oxford Dictionary of English Etymology.* Oxford: Clarendon Press.

Persch, A.C., Pizur-Barnekow, K., Cashin, S., & Pickens, N.D. (2009). Heart rate variability of activity and occupation during solitary and social engagement. *Journal of Occupational Science,* **16**, 163–9.

Pierce, D., Atler, K., Baltisberger, J. *et al.* (2010). Occupational science: A data-based American perspective. *Journal of Occupational Science,* **17**, 204–15.

Sampson, R., & Gifford, S.M. (2010). Place-making, settlement and well-being: The therapeutic landscapes of recently arrived youth with refugee backgrounds. *Health & Place,* **16**, 116–31. doi:10.1016/j.healthplace.2009.09.004

Simpson, J.A., & Weiner, E.S.C. (Eds). (1989). *The Oxford English Dictionary* (2nd ed., Vol. XIV). Oxford: Clarendon Press.

Steckler, A., & Linnan, L. (Eds). (2002). *Process Evaluation for Public Health Interventions and Research.* San Francisco: Jossey-Bass.

UNESCO. (2010). United Nations Educational, Scientific and Cultural Organization. *Building Peace in the Minds of Men and Women.* Retrieved from http://www.unesco.org/new/en/unesco/about-us/who-we-are/introducing-unesco/(last accessed 25 June 2011).

UNHCR Division of Programme Support and Management. (2010). *2009 Global Trends: Refugees, Asylum-seekers, Returnees, Internally Displaced and Stateless Persons.* Geneva: United Nations High Commissioner for Refugees.

UNHCR: The UN Refugee Agency. (2010). *Resettlement.* Retrieved from http://www.unhcr.org/pages/4a16b1676.html (last accessed 25 June 2011).

United Nations (UN). (2010). *United Nations: We the peoples ... A stronger UN for a better world.* Retrieved from http://www.un.org/en/index.shtml (last accessed 25 June 2011).

UN Department of Economic and Social Affairs. (2009). *World Population Ageing 1950–2050.* Retrieved from http://www.un.org/esa/population/publications/worldageing19502050/ (last accessed 25 June 2011).

UN Programme on Ageing. (2007). *Research Agenda on Ageing for the 21st Century: A Joint Project of the United Nations Programme on Ageing and the International Association of Gerontology and Geriatrics.* Retrieved from http://www.un.org/ageing/documents/AgeingResearchAgenda-6.pdf (last accessed 25 June 2011).

Wilcock, A.A. (1993). A theory of the human need for occupation. *Journal of Occupational Science,* **1**, 17–24.

Wilcock, A.A. (2003). A science of occupation: Ancient or modern. *Journal of Occupational Science: Australia,* **10**, 115–19.

Wood, W., Womack, J., & Hooper, B. (2009). Dying of boredom: An exploratory case study of time use, apparent affect, and routine activity situations on two Alzheimer's special care units. *American Journal of Occupational Therapy,* **63**, 337–50.

World Health Organization (WHO). (2010). *The WHO agenda.* Retrieved from http://www.who.int/about/agenda/en/index.html (last accessed 25 June 2011).

Worldwatch Institute. (2008). *Vital Signs: Global Trends that Shape our Future.* Retrieved from http://vitalsigns.worldwatch.org/ (last accessed 25 June 2011).

Yerxa, E.J. (1998). Health and the human spirit for occupation. *American Journal of Occupational Therapy*, **52**, 412–18.
Yerxa, E.J., Clark, F., Frank, G. *et al.* (1989). An introduction to occupational science: A foundation for occupational therapy in the 21st century. *Occupational Therapy in Health Care*, **6**, 1–17.
Zemke, R., & Clark, F. (1996). Preface. In R. Zemke & F. Clark (Eds), *Occupational Science: The Evolving Discipline* (pp. vii–xviii). Philadelphia, PA: F.A. Davis.

11

Occupational choice: The significance of socio-economic and political factors

Roshan Galvaan

An enabling approach to occupational justice is premised on the understanding that humans choose to engage in occupations. Choosing occupations, however, is a complex, socio-culturally situated matter: at any moment what an individual chooses to do is influenced by a myriad of factors ranging from the individual (such as skills levels) to the extrapersonal (such as resource availability). Accordingly, issues of equity of access and justice need to be acknowledged in any discussion of what constitutes occupational choice and how it can best be understood. In this chapter I draw on my critical ethnographic study describing young adolescents' occupational choices in a marginalized community in Cape Town, South Africa (Galvaan, 2010). I discuss the intersecting socio-economic and political influences that contribute to young adolescents making hegemonic occupational choices which maintain historically predicated patterns and perpetuate occupational injustice. I conclude by articulating the dynamic ways in which socio-economic and political contexts influence occupational choice to both constrain and enable participation.

When considering occupational justice, it is important to acknowledge the central tenet that 'humans participate as autonomous, yet interdependent agents in their social contexts' and that 'empowerment depends on enabling choice and control in occupational participation' (Townsend & Wilcock, 2004, p. 79). Choices include making decisions about and between occupations. The concept of occupational justice emphasizes an individual's choice in accepting opportunities and resources that support their enablement

Occupational Science: Society, Inclusion, Participation, First Edition.
Edited by Gail Whiteford and Clare Hocking.

and empowerment (Townsend & Whiteford, 2004). The underlying assumption is that the right and power to exert preferences exists and that perceptions of choice and control are influenced by social and cultural dimensions (Townsend & Wilcock, 2004). This is particularly significant for marginalized groups since their rights and power to exert preferences related to occupations may not exist. Occupational injustice may thus arise from a lack of occupational choice; as such, understanding more about occupational choice may reveal ways to promote occupational justice for marginalized groups.

Critical ethnographic research exploring occupational choice

Young adolescents living in the community of Lavender Hill are one such example of a marginalized group. In 2010, I conducted a critical ethnography of these adolescents' occupational choices, which are best understood through the socio-historical context of the research.

Lavender Hill is an area on the Cape Flats in the Southern Peninsula of Cape Town, South Africa. This area was constructed between 1972 and 1974 under the South African Group Areas Act of 1950, which proclaimed that people from different racial groups should live in separate areas according to their designated races; Lavender Hill had been zoned as a coloured residential area. (Under apartheid, 'coloured' was one of the race classifications, referring to people of mixed descent.) Instead of the legitimized, objectified construction of race associated with apartheid, race is viewed here as a social, rather than biological category which is constructed and can be deconstructed and challenged. It is associated with material power and privilege. Race conditions in South Africa form part of people's daily experiences (Distiller & Steyn, 2004), and coloured identity, which also represents a creolized identity, continues to evolve (Erasmus, 2001a).

Coloured people were forcibly moved from prestigious areas close to central business districts with recreation facilities and resources to remote areas without infrastructure. Many had previously been property owners, but were forced to sell their property for very little and could not afford to buy in the areas they were relocated to (Naidoo & Dreyer, 1984). For many of the people moved to Lavender Hill, housing rental costs increased. The area remains characterized by poverty and community violence, lack of opportunities or services for youth, gangsterism and drug abuse. People live in overcrowded conditions, lack access to social services and have poor access to formal recreational opportunities. Statistical socio-economic indicators have reflected high levels of unemployment, and low income and educational levels in Lavender Hill (StatsSA, 2001).

My study explored the occupational choices of seven young adolescent participants in Lavender Hill. Critical ethnographic methods of inquiry were applied over four years with data gathering consisting of photovoice methods and photo-elicitation interviews based on photographs that participants had taken, followed by participant observation sessions. Interviews were also conducted with participants and their parents or guardians. The data analyses led to findings that identified the nature of and influences on the participants' occupational choices. As a result, occupational choice was defined as follows:

> *Occupational choice involves the application of choice to participation in occupations; occupational choices are co-constructed through their transactional*

relationship with the context. An occupational choice can be made, manifesting as a process. It is also an outcome of a decision relating to participation in occupations. It occurs implicitly and explicitly when agency is applied to occupational engagement. (adapted from Galvaan, 2010, p. vi)

The occupational choices made by the research participants emerged as inextricably linked with the context. Lavender Hill did more than serve as a backdrop for occupational choice; instead it became part of occupational choice, contributing to creating occupational choice. Within the context, the factors influencing occupational choice included the young adolescents' experiences of the historically predicated patterns of occupations at a community level in Lavender Hill, the subcultures of subgroups, the competition for forms of capital, and the low educational expectations held of them. These factors did not function in a binary fashion. Instead, they influenced occupational choice in a composite manner and intersected with each other. Insight into the relationship between (social) structure and (human) agency in shaping social action (Bourdieu, 1977) is helpful in shedding light on the reasons for occupational choice, since occupation is a form of social action. Context is perceived as corresponding to the social structures and processes, with young adolescents as the agents making occupational choices. The following section focuses upon and explains the particular way in which socio-economic and political factors shaped the patterns of young adolescents' occupational choices in Lavender Hill.

Socio-economic and political influences on occupational choice

It was clear that the occupational choices of the young adolescents in Lavender Hill were always influenced by the past. They were contingent upon, and consistent with, those historic socio-economic and politically asserted patterns of occupational engagement that have developed and been perpetuated in Lavender Hill since apartheid. The participants made occupational choices by considering the limited range of occupations already available in their context, and to which they had been exposed. Socio-economic and political influences were present in the social structures within which occupational choice occurred, and the available physical structures shaped the young adolescents' dispositions, while their discourse and linguistic expressions perpetuated their historically predicated patterns. These factors are explained below.

Physical structures contribute to a disposition of limited available occupations

The people who were relocated to Lavender Hill were placed in apartment-style housing or *kortse*, where the way of living reflected components of coloured identity. The association of the kortse historically with apartheid and continually with coloured culture was evident within the study, and at a community level, the young adolescents who participated positioned themselves as part of this coloured community. They associated their occupational choices with the lifestyle of people living in housing structures such as the kortse or *hokkies* (little shacks) that all of the participants experienced living in for periods of their lives. They accepted these structures as a normal way of life for themselves and fellow community members. Living in the kortse and informal dwellings left them making occupational choices based on what they knew to be happening in the physical spaces with which they were familiar. Their choices were influenced on a daily basis by the substandard housing and communal recreation structures that have not changed significantly since apartheid.

The young adolescents' experiences showed the effects of the historical legacy of no planning for the expansion of the area. This resulted in their acceptance of this standard of living as part of their day-to-day experiences. The depth of the participants' involvement in the realities shaping their homes (such as parents abusing alcohol or sparse living conditions) emerged in relation to their occupational choices. While this sometimes had a direct influence, the substandard living conditions and associated culture were normative and thus, for young adolescents living in Lavender Hill, continuously framed their dispositions, which in turn informed their occupational choices.

An earlier ethnographic study conducted by Salo (2004) in Manenberg, an area on the Cape Flats similar to Lavender Hill, also highlighted the influence of the kortse way of life. She indicated that the lifestyle associated with living in the kortse shaped the way that personhood was experienced. Similarly, young adolescents in Lavender Hill showed an awareness of the evolved behavioural and social rules associated with living there. For example, participants described knowing that gang signs could be used as a mechanism to protect themselves, explaining that their hand signs were symbols showing their identification, not membership of the notorious Cape Flats Americans gang. This identification did not mean that they were gang members or that they explicitly aspired to become part of the gangs. When explaining why they showed gang signs, one explanation given was so that they would not be seen as the opposition and thus as a threat by the gangsters. Being viewed as non-threatening served to protect them from possible harm. Additionally, showing the signs signified compliance and respect for the gangs and gangsters. It was held as positive social status, and was seen as cool. These explanations were presented concurrently and were equally cogent for the participants. Overall, the young adolescents' interpretations and compliance with the variety of known behavioural and social rules influenced their occupational choices.

Socio-economic class contributes to the predicated patterns

Lavender Hill is a characteristically working-class community (StatsSA, 2001) historically associated with the coloured preferential labour policy (people classified as black under apartheid legislation were not readily allowed into areas such as Lavender Hill). The lived experiences of the young adolescents and the tacit knowledge that they drew on in making occupational choices were congruent with viewing themselves as rooted in such a community. Their acceptance of the economic limitations impacted on their interpretation of occupations and opportunities, and they predominantly considered themselves as participating in the occupations they saw others in their communities doing.

This was evident in their comfortable association with being part of the manual labour workforce, or positions requiring minimal or no education and training. They appeared to be marginalized as part of a lower income, working-class community which perpetuated the marginalization introduced during apartheid.

Patterns of occupations that were common in the community, such as dropping out of school, appeared synonymous with this disposition for young adolescents in Lavender Hill. Consequently, their occupational choices perpetuated patterns of participation that reflected historic socio-cultural norms. Their occupational choices resulted in similar trajectories to previous generations, with identity constructions evidencing an ideological continuity with the way that coloured identity was constructed during apartheid. This extended to the participants' perspectives of the limited achievements possible for coloured youth. They did not see opportunities to make different occupational choices, or when alternative occupational choices were identified, these were seen as inaccessible. When explicitly seeking to engage in occupations, the participants weighed up options and scanned the environment for opportunities. It was evident that their decisions to engage in occupations depended on their expectations and prior experiences of the occupations. Adults served as role models despite the adolescents explicitly disapproving of some of the adults' behaviours. The contradiction in participants' occupational choices was that they sometimes made occupational choices similar to the adults in the community of whom they disapproved. The following example from a participant illustrates this.

Alcohol, like (tobacco) cigarettes was part of the everyday routine of many adults in Lavender Hill. Some participants disapproved of the daily use of alcohol. A participant expressed his disappointment in his mother:

> *Participant 1: Daar gaan nie dinge reg aan nie... my Ma sy drink nou 'n dop, my Ma, nou so is dit.*
> (Participant 1: The things that are going on are not right... my mother takes a tot, that is how it is.)

He recognized the reality that alcohol abuse was part of his daily experience whilst reflecting on its essential 'not right-edness' – perhaps indicating a desire for difference but an inability to affect such change. The negative impact of alcohol misuse on daily life was also felt by another participant who described looking after his younger sister when his mother was drunk. Furthermore, the participants conveyed their familiarity with illegal shebeens since they had all, on many previous occasions, been sent to one to buy beer for an adult. Because alcohol use was normative, people in the neighbourhood who saw young adolescents carrying alcohol did not question it. Furthermore, young adolescents indulged in tasting it, despite experiencing the negative consequences of the adults' continued consumption. A participant described an incident during a visit to Uncle Dirkie's game shop when he was seven years old.

> *Participant 2: My Ma-hulle het daar gesit en gedrink, toe speel ek net games. Toe speel ek eerste lekker toe sien ek hier begin die mense te baklei, toe steek die man vir die vrou hier by die kant, regdeur, amper dood...*
> *Researcher: Sjoe.*

Participant 2: Klomp bloed ook uitgetap. Toe hardloop my Ma uit met my uit.

(Participant 2: My mother sat there drinking (alcohol) and I was just playing games. So I was first enjoying playing and then I saw people starting to fight, so the man stabbed the woman here on the side, almost right through, almost dead ...

Researcher: Wow.

Participant 2: A whole lot of blood gushed out. So my mother ran out with me.)

This participant witnessed how the people that his mother associated with were arguing and then physically fighting. He expressed his disapproval of his mother visiting the game shop and using alcohol, and did not view her as a good role model. When participants cited examples of adults misbehaving in this way, they questioned why they should listen to those adults. These questions were not often posed as explicit challenges, possibly because of their respect for – and fear of – adults. Adding to the normalization of alcohol use was that the illegal shebeens and games shops were often on the same property. The implication of this was that while a participant played at the games shop, adults may have been abusing alcohol close by. Consequently young adolescents were exposed to the adult occupation of drinking alcohol while they were playing. The irony of the participants' occupational choices lay in the tension between those choices and what they professed as the right thing to choose. Further to this, the adults who disagreed with the adolescents' occupational choices seemed unable to take positive action to change them.

Consistent with the parents' inert stance relative to the adolescents' needs was their apparent lack of attention to 'homework'. Although the parents tried their best to preach the importance of schooling to children, that value was not evident in the structures they put in place to enable or support the young adolescents' academic achievement. Instead, adults commonly condoned corporal punishment as a strategy for enforcing their message, which seemed to have limited impact on the occupational choices that youth made. In keeping with the disjunction between their parents' espoused values and actions, and the low expectations placed upon them, the participants in this study attended school but their academic efforts were minimal.

Their occupational choices emerged from their local lived experiences, which in turn shaped their occupational patterns. The participants progressively aligned both their view of possibilities and their actions with what they saw happening for others in the community, even though they might still have had the hope of achieving more. Consequently their trajectories framed the way the participants perceived and approached opportunities. The importance of the way that social structures shape and are shaped by everyday living is recognized in sociology and occupational therapy. Social structures play a part in producing agency in social life and this agency contributes to creating the structures (Cuff, Sharrock, & Francis, 2006). Applying this insight to occupational choice emphasizes its relational, transactional nature. Occupational choice may be seen as a mechanism contributing to agency and through this, creating social structures. That is, through making occupational choices, young adolescents exercise their agency and contribute to social structures. The discourse associated with occupational choice is an important ideological and operational aspect of the production of occupational choice and is elaborated upon below.

Discourse and linguistic expression perpetuates the predicated patterns

The occupational choices that the young adolescents made were communicated using the language of *gamtaal*. Gamtaal is a Cape Flats dialect of Afrikaans, which is considered to reflect a working-class coloured identity (Haupt, 2001). The participants persistently used gamtaal to identify, describe and explain their occupational choices. Common phrases such as being *wys* or sussed expressed a way of knowing how things are done in a coloured community. Historically, gamtaal was accepted by coloured communities and others as being socially inferior (Adhikari, 2005) and this subversively persists despite South Africa's policy of multilingualism. This is of concern as the English language has become part of a wider institutional and societal discourse, where it holds powerful status and influences possible social mobility (Kapp, 2006). The reality for some Xhosa-speaking young adolescents was that they did not have the choice of learning in their mother tongue in Lavender Hill. It appeared that they had to assimilate to using predominantly gamtaal. This manifested the ongoing impact of Lavender Hill's designation as a coloured racial preferential area under the Group Areas Act. Politics are thus salient in shaping the contribution of the language used to communicate, and arguably, also to construct occupational choices.

The language used by young adolescents constructed their occupational choices contributed to the perpetuation of the hegemony of historically predicated patterns. This implies that the historical patterns of occupational choices are ever present in the construction of current occupational choices. This suggestion is supported by the view that coloured identity is distinctively shaped and reshaped in the contexts of slavery, colonialism and cultural dispossession, which leaves its constructed and composite historical nature always evident and dislocation always present (Erasmus, 2001b). As evidenced in the participants' discourse, the occupational choices for young adolescents in Lavender Hill perpetuated the hegemony of being part of a coloured working-class community.

Further to this, their views of the occupational choices possible for them in the future were limited to those opportunities that they knew to be readily available in Lavender Hill. This resulted in a restricted mindset with which to consider making occupational choices.

Occupational choice as a contributor to occupational engagement

Recognizing that occupational engagement is a form of social action that occurs in multiple contexts leads to a perspective that can transcend the duality between person and environment (Dickie, Cutchin, & Humphry, 2006). This perspective re-theorized occupation from a less individualized orientation, with Dickie, Cutchin and Humphry (2006) asserting that drawing on Dewey and Bourdieu's action theories re-orientates occupation as transactional. From that perspective, context and occupational engagement are co-constructions and occupation is seen as the relational glue between the person and his or her environment (Cutchin *et al.*, 2008). Based on the research findings reported above, I propose that occupational choice is a mediating factor that may contribute to the relationship between the person and the environment. Bourdieu's theory of social practice (Bourdieu, 1977, 1990) can assist in grasping how this may be possible.

Bourdieu (1977) acknowledged the importance of both the individual and the society in shaping human action and creating social structure. He explained that society shapes individuals through socialization, but that the continuity of society depends on the individual's actions (Bourdieu, 1990). Since occupations are forms of social action (Cutchin *et al.*, 2008), it is asserted that the patterns of occupations over time contribute to the continuity of society. Based on my study, I contend that occupational choice gives rise to occupations, thus it is possible that occupational choices over time result in occupations that contribute to the continuity of society. Bourdieu (1977) identified three interrelated concepts, namely habitus, capital and social field (Jenkins, 1992), which have to be grasped in order to understand how choices can be viewed as social practice. For the purposes of the current chapter, only habitus is introduced as it is most pertinent to conceptualizing occupational choice.

Bourdieu strongly criticized rational choice theory (Reed-Danahay, 2005). The intention here is not to contribute to the debate of the conceptualization of choice. Rather, it is accepted that choice exists and that its existence transcends functioning at a rational level. Instead choice is viewed with respect to the relationship between social structure and humans as agents (Bourdieu, 1977, 1990). Bourdieu (1990) proposed that choices are made under the constraints of habitus and the conditions of social fields. Habitus refers to a semi-conscious orientation that humans have to the world (Jenkins, 1992). This orientation is shaped by the context and inclines people to act in particular ways (Bourdieu, 1990). This implies that particular choices are made within a specific context.

Applied to the young adolescents in Lavender Hill, it means that they developed particular orientations or dispositions that influenced their occupational engagement and inclined them to make particular occupational choices. Habitus emerges from an embodied history that is internalized as second nature and is active as the whole past of which it is a product (Bourdieu, 1990). People's dispositions generate actions that are regular, but not consciously governed by rules; actions are governed by the social positions that people hold. This is likened to the idiosyncratic, yet patterned nature of occupation, since occupations are not only influenced by habits but also contribute to the formation of habits (Cutchin *et al.*, 2008). Furthermore, it is advocated that habitus is not individual, but is shared by a collective holding similar positions (Bourdieu, 1990), for example young adolescents in the same social class in Lavender Hill. The past, as part of habitus, functions as accumulated capital and produces history based in history. This process may contribute to the consistency of occupational engagement for particular groups across history, since habitus is transposable and generative.

The young adolescents' construction of occupational choice appeared as contextually bound. That is, the context and occupational choice seemed inseparable. Likewise, social structure does not exist independently of human agency since agents interact with social structures to fulfil norms that fit their images of what reality is (Cassell, 1993). In relation to occupational choice, young adolescents' dispositions may leave them inclined to generate occupational choices consistent with their social positions. It means that although an individual may have access to many opportunities, those options may not be reflected in their occupational choices. This may be as a consequence of the interaction between human agency and social structures. An individual's agency may play a further role in the selection process, since occupational choice occurs during and prior to occupational performance (Galvaan, 2010). Depending on an individual's experience of participating in an occupation and the occupational choices made during occupational performance, he or she might make decisions about how to further exert agency. In this way, agency expressed during and through occupational performance might also shape ongoing occupational choices. It is proposed that occupational choice may be one mechanism whereby agents and structures define and reproduce each other.

Viewing occupational choice as a mechanism contributing to agency and social structure holds implications for occupational science and occupational therapy. It adds credence to the belief that occupation is central to health, well-being and human development (Christiansen, Baum, & Bass-Haugen, 2005). Contributing to the enactment of human agency, the transactional relationship between occupational choice and social structure is advocated as a core contributor to the essential nature of occupation. The influence of socio-economic and political factors on occupational choice also supports the assertion that underlying occupational determinants shape occupational engagement and may lead to occupational risk considerations. The implications of this for the way that occupational therapists approach their work with marginalized groups, such as the young adolescents in Lavender Hill, is that more focus should be given to underlying occupational determinants in terms of their everyday contribution to shaping occupational choice.

The invisible, normative standardization of low expectations for occupational engagement (Townsend & Wilcock, 2004), as revealed by the young adolescents' occupational choices in Lavender Hill, is a feature of occupational marginalization. Access to a diverse range of occupations (Polatajko *et al.*, 2007) has been promoted as key to overcoming occupational marginalization. However, merely introducing diverse occupations is not sufficient to facilitate social change. It is argued that, in addition to introducing opportunities to engage in diverse occupational choices, the hegemonic manner in which occupational choices may traditionally have been made has to be addressed. This involves identifying emerging patterns of occupational choices. A critical analysis of the patterns of occupational choice can uncover the ways in which underlying occupational determinants surface.

Conclusion

This chapter, through the presentation of research findings, has illuminated the highly situated nature of occupational choice. It has discussed the multiple ways in which historical and prevailing socio-economic and political factors may influence individuals' occupational choices. In particular, the transactional relationship between context and occupational choice and the implications this has for promoting occupational justice has been explored as a basis for transformative practice.

References

Adhikari, M. (2005). *Not White Enough, Not Black Enough: Racial Identity in the South African Coloured Community*. Athens: Ohio University Press.

Bourdieu, P. (1977). *Outline of a Theory of Practice* (trans. R. Nice). Cambridge: Cambridge University Press.

Bourdieu, P. (1990). *The Logic of Practice* (trans. R. Nice). Cambridge: Polity Press.

Cassell, P. (1993). *The Giddens Reader*. London: Macmillan.

Christiansen, C.H., Baum, C.M., & Bass-Haugen, J. (2005). *Occupational Therapy: Performance, Participation and Wellbeing*. Thorofare: Slack.

Cuff, E., Sharrock, W., & Francis, D. (2006). *Perspectives in Sociology* (5th ed.) New York: Routledge.

Cutchin, M.P., Aldrich, R.M., Baillard, A.L., & Coppola, S. (2008). Action theories for occupational science: The contributions of Dewey and Bourdieu. *Journal of Occupational Science*, **15**, 157–64.

Dickie, V., Cutchin, M.P., & Humphry, R. (2006). Occupation as transactional experience: A critique of individualism in occupational science. *Journal of Occupational Science*, **13**, 83–93.

Distiller, N., & Steyn, M. (2004). *Under Construction: 'Race' and Identity in South Africa Today*. Sandton: Heinemann Publishers.

Erasmus, Z. (2001a). *Coloured by History, Shaped by Place: New Perspectives on Coloured Identities in Cape Town*. Cape Town: Kwela Books.

Erasmus, Z. (2001b). Re-imagining coloured identities in post-apartheid South Africa. In Z. Erasmus (Ed.), *Coloured by History, Shaped by Place: New Perspectives on Coloured Identities in Cape Town* (pp. 13–28). Cape Town: Kwela Books.

Galvaan, R. (2010). *A critical ethnography of young adolescents' occupational choices in a community in post-apartheid South Africa*. PhD thesis, University of Cape Town, Cape Town.

Haupt, A. (2001). Black thing: Hip hop nationalism race and gender in Prophets of da City and Brasse Vannie Kaap. In Z. Erasmus (Ed.), *Coloured by History, Shaped by Place: New Perspectives on Coloured Identities in Cape Town* (pp. 173–91). Cape Town: Kwela Books.

Jenkins, R. (1992). *Pierre Bourdieu*. London: Routledge.

Kapp, R. (2006). Discourses of English and literacy in a Western Cape township school. In L. Thesen & E.V. Pletzen (Eds), *Academic Literacy and the Languages of Change* (pp. 30–52). London: Continuum.

Naidoo, W., & Dreyer, W. (1984). *Area Study of Vrygrond and Lavender Hill*. Paper presented at the Carnegie Conference Paper No.10b, Cape Town.

Polatajko, H., Molke, D., Baptiste, S. *et al.* (2007). Social context and occupational choice from the perspective of Brenda Beagan and Zofia Kumas-Tan. In E.A. Townsend & H.J. Polatajko (Eds), *Enabling Occupation II: Advancing an Occupational Therapy Vision for Health, Well-being and Justice through Occupation* (pp. 72–4). Ottawa: Canadian Association of Occupational Therapists, ACE.

Reed-Danahay, D. (2005). *Locating Bourdieu*. Bloomington: Indiana University Press.

Salo, E. (2004). *Respectable Mothers, Tough Men and Good Daughters*. Unpublished Doctoral Dissertation, University of Cape Town, Cape Town.
South African Group Areas Act. (Act No 41 of 1950).
StatsSA. (2001). *Statistics South Africa – Census 2001*.
Townsend, E., & Whiteford, G. (2004). A participatory occupational justice framework: Population-based processes of practice. In F. Kronenberg, S.S. Algado & N. Pollard (Eds), *Occupational Therapy without Borders: Learning from the Spirit of Survivors* (pp. 110–26). London: Elsevier.
Townsend, E., & Wilcock, A. (2004). Occupational justice and client-centred practice: A dialogue in progress. *Canadian Journal of Occupational Therapy*, **71**, 75–87.

12

The International Society for Occupational Science: A critique of its role in facilitating the development of occupational science through international networks and intercultural dialogue

Alison Wicks

The real world

At 3:34 a.m. local time, 27 February 2010, a devastating magnitude 8.8 earthquake struck Chile, one of the strongest earthquakes ever recorded. An estimated 2 million people were affected in some way by damage to infrastructure such as highways and airports, and forced closure of shops, businesses and schools. The resultant occupational disruption in communities and impact on the daily routines of the Chilean people was massive. A year later, coastal communities in Japan were devastated by a magnitude 9.0 earthquake and the associated tidal wave that swept away buildings, boats and cars, and wrought havoc on a Japanese nuclear power plant.

Occupational Science: Society, Inclusion, Participation, First Edition.
Edited by Gail Whiteford and Clare Hocking.

Every day around the world people's daily lives are disrupted by natural disasters and wars. In many countries, people suffer occupational injustices from government policies and socio-cultural mores. Individual and community health and well-being are negatively impacted as a result.

The dream

An occupational perspective is mainstream, incorporated into government policies and programmes to promote participation and community development, especially for those suffering occupational injustices. It is widely acknowledged that for health and well- being, people and communities need opportunities to do things that are personally and culturally relevant. ISOS is a well-known, respected and financially viable international society representing national occupational science societies and related groups. It manages programmes facilitating collaboration in occupational science education and research, and promoting occupational science around the world. It is a peak body advocating occupational justice.

The International Society for Occupational Science (ISOS) is a virtual society advocating for an occupationally just world, a world in which people have opportunities and choices to do the things they need and want to do. Its current mission is the facilitation of a worldwide network of individuals and institutions committed to research and education on occupation and to the promotion of engagement in occupation for health and community development. Over the past 10 years, ISOS has made some significant contributions to the international development of occupational science and has informed people around the world about the existence of occupational science, its relationship to practice, and its potential to shape policy by promoting how occupational engagement impacts on health and well-being. Yet, today, an occupational perspective is rarely adopted when addressing the broad lifestyle issues confronting the twenty-first century. So how can ISOS realize its vision and spark the occupational imagination of urban planners, politicians and practitioners? This chapter explores ways in which ISOS can be developed in a sustainable way to achieve its goals and uphold its principles of inclusion and diversity whilst developing a unified vision.

Since 1999, a team of volunteers from around the world have coordinated ISOS activities. I have been actively involved since its inception, initially as an assistant for the Inaugural ISOS Board, and since 2007 as a member of the Board. I also have maintained an archive of ISOS correspondence and documents which has been a useful resource for this chapter. Consequently, I have a unique insider's knowledge and understanding of decisions made and strategies implemented over the past decade, enabling me to reflect on the progress of ISOS. My primary aim in writing this chapter is to critically evaluate the contributions ISOS has made to the international occupational science community through the various activities it has undertaken and the vision it has developed for the future of occupational science. The second aim is to document some important milestones in the ISOS story and provide insight into its trajectory. The comments in this chapter have been shaped by my discussions with others who have also been closely involved in ISOS and the development of occupational science.

This chapter begins with an overview of the global spread of occupational science during the past 20 years and a synopsis of the ISOS story, to contextualize the discussion that follows on the ideological frameworks which have structured and supported the ISOS mission and strategic plan. Examples of the contributions ISOS has made to the development of resources and strategies to enable individuals and institutions to stay informed of developments in occupational science, as well as to make links with others who share similar interests, are presented next. The chapter concludes with reflections on the challenges of growing a virtual international society in a sustainable way and proposals to ensure that ISOS promotes occupational science's potential to positively influence policy, practice and people's participation.

The development of occupational science internationally

Occupational science has been developing in countries all around the world, in different ways and at different rates since its genesis in the late 1980s. At that time, post-modernism was fostering awareness of questions about power and diversity and fuelling interest in new ways of knowing, such as the interpretive sciences (Whiteford, Townsend, & Hocking, 2000). Concurrently, the profession of occupational therapy was purportedly experiencing intra-professional challenges and grappling with an identity crisis (Kielhofner, 1997). From these post-modern and professional issues arose a paradigm of thought focused on occupation which has been referred to as 'an occupational renaissance' (Whiteford *et al.*, 2000, p. 62). A team of academics, consisting primarily of occupational therapists but also an anthropologist and psychologist, responded to this occupational renaissance by identifying the need for a science of occupation, not only as a theoretical foundation for occupational therapy, but also to provide evidence for practice. Interestingly, these founders maintained that occupational science needed contributions from a wide variety of disciplines in order to understand occupation, which they acknowledged as a very complex phenomenon (Wilcock, 1991; Yerxa, 1989). However, creating an interdisciplinary science has been challenging (Molineux & Whiteford, 2005) and by 2000, 10 years after its establishment, occupational therapists were still the large majority of published authors in the field of occupational science (Molke, Laliberte Rudman, & Polatajko, 2004).

Although other professions and disciplines are yet to embrace occupational science, key occupational therapy leaders have supported the global spread and increasing recognition of occupational science. The renaming of occupational therapy education programmes in Australia, Canada, Ireland, New Zealand and the United States to include occupational science attests to the perceived quality of research and scholarship in the field. Occupational science is an identified focus of the European Network of Occupational Therapists (ENOTHE), a collaboration of occupational therapy schools across Europe, and supporters of occupational science were instrumental in giving occupation prominence in the World Federation of Occupational Therapists' (2002) Minimum Standards for the Education of Occupational Therapists. Degree programmes in occupational science are offered in the United States and Japan. The *Journal of Occupational Science* (JOS), established in 1993 to promote the study of humans as occupational beings, supports these educational programmes by publishing peer reviewed feature articles by authors from around the world. JOS increased its number of annual issues from three to four in 2010, an indication of the growing number of occupational science scholars writing for publication. Additionally, national occupational science groups have been emerging around the world over the last 10 years. Today, there are groups in Australasia, Canada, Chile, Japan, the United Kingdom and Ireland, and the United States (Clark & Lawlor, 2009). The most recently established occupational science group is in Brazil (Otavio Folha, personal communication, October 2010).

These occupational science groups, which vary in size and function, are continually evolving to meet member needs and address issues as they emerge within the field. There are commonalities and differences with regard to their missions in respect to occupational science. For example, since September 2000, the Australasian Society of Occupational Scientists (ASOS) has been facilitating 'an Australasian network of individuals and institutions committed to research and education on occupation' (ASOS, n.d.). The mission of the Canadian Society of Occupational Scientists (CSOS), formed in May 2001, is to build 'a Canadian, interdisciplinary organization to coordinate interests in occupational science and promote its continued growth' (CSOS, 2010). The mission of the Society for the Study of Occupation: United States of America (SSO:USA), is 'to facilitate high quality scholarship and a dynamic exchange of ideas that support the discipline' (SSO:USA, 2005).

The Division of Occupational Science and Occupational Therapy at the University of Southern California (USC), headed by Dr Florence Clark, has hosted annual occupational science symposia since 1989, the 22nd symposium being held in 2010. The national societies and other relevant associations have followed the lead established by USC by also holding symposia. JOS hosted the first Australasian symposium in 1997, while OccupationUK held its first symposium in York, in 1999. There have been occupational science symposia in Japan for the past 14 years, even though the Japanese Society for the Study of Occupation was not formed until November 2006. Since it was formally established in November 2002, SSO:USA has conducted annual symposia throughout the USA to share and showcase research in occupation. CSOS has been hosting biennial occupational science symposia since 2002 as well. The Chilean Society for the Study of Occupation held its first symposium in 2009. Occupational science symposia and workshops have been held in Taiwan and Europe in recent years.

While the national societies and groups have been developing over the past decade, there has been a concomitant epistemic development in occupational science internationally. In the beginning, the primary discourse was on occupation for health, not surprising perhaps given the founders of the science were primarily health professionals. However, currently, a new discourse on occupational participation as a human right is being embraced, as demonstrated at the Joint CSOS–SSO:USA Conference held in October 2010 where the keynote speakers guided discussion on justice and advocacy issues. The changing foci, purpose and methods in occupational science studies, as revealed by recent analyses (Glover, 2009; Pierce *et al.*, 2010) seemingly reflect the changing discourse. As an additional consequence, proponents of occupational science are being challenged to consider new theories, such as complexity theory (Whiteford, Klomp, & Wright-St Clair, 2005) and new perspectives, such as a transactional view of occupation (Dickie, Cutchin, & Humphry, 2006). Resultant tension and disjuncture arising from epistemic development are part of the maturation of occupational science.

This overview of the international development of occupational science, which has highlighted its global spread and identified key issues that are influencing the future direction of occupational science, helps to contextualize the following brief history of ISOS and explain its raison d'être and the key determinants that have shaped its story since 1999. Additional historical details are available on the ISOS website (ISOS, 2009).

A brief history of ISOS

In April 1999, at the Occupational Therapy Australia Conference in Canberra, 28 Australians, 3 New Zealanders and 1 Canadian attended a meeting to discuss a proposal to establish an international group for the study of humans as occupational beings. This proposal, put forward by Ann Wilcock, originated from discussions among delegates at the 1998 World Federation of Occupational Therapists (WFOT) Congress in Montreal. At that congress, a presentation by Wilcock (1998) on the role of an occupational perspective in addressing individual, community and environmental needs, which highlighted the occupational foundations of the Ottawa Charter for Health Promotion (WHO, 1986), stimulated ideas about a broader agenda for occupational therapy. Of particular relevance to the 1999 meeting in Australia and the subsequent focus of ISOS is that many of those at the meeting had attended a conference workshop on occupational justice convened by Ann Wilcock and Elizabeth Townsend. Townsend, the sole Canadian at the meeting, was invited to the conference as a keynote speaker. Hence, ideas about equity and human rights were 'in the air'.

The attendees of that Canberra meeting not only supported Wilcock's proposal to establish an international occupational science group, but immediately proceeded to form the International Interdisciplinary Group for the Promotion of Occupational Science (IIGPOS). They also agreed to develop a proposal for WFOT support of the group. A working party comprised of volunteers from the Canberra meeting and invited international representatives subsequently developed and submitted the proposal to WFOT and then responded to questions as to how IIGPOS could best interact with WFOT which, at that time, was about to introduce programme management to its organizational structure.

The outcomes of these deliberations between the working party and WFOT were threefold. The first outcome was the decision that IIGPOS would be separate from WFOT to encourage members from various professions, not just occupational therapy, thereby promoting interdisciplinarity in occupational science. Second, it was decided to rename the group as the International Society of Occupational Scientists. A third outcome was a proposal to establish WFOT International Advisory Groups with the International Advisory Group in Occupational Science (IAG:OS) being the pilot group. This proposal recognized the relationship between occupational science and occupational therapy, acknowledged the support of WFOT for occupational science and provided a means of keeping WFOT informed of developments in occupational science that were specifically relevant to occupational therapy. The proposal for the IAG:OS was endorsed by the WFOT Council in Japan in 2000. Although an initiative of the society, the advisory group and society have always had different terms of reference

Table 12.1 ISOS Mission Statement, 2000

Vision

By 2005, there will be a worldwide network of occupational scientists across diverse disciplines and interested groups and organizations advocating occupational justice for world health and well-being.

Mission

The International Society of Occupational Scientists (ISOS) aims to advance world health, well-being and justice by energizing a worldwide network of individuals, groups and organizations to research, debate and activate for equity of opportunity for people, according to an understanding of their occupational nature.

Four key beliefs underlie ISOS. They are:

1. Occupation encompasses all human pursuits; mental, physical, social and spiritual; restful, reflective and active; obligatory or self-chosen; paid or unpaid.
2. Occupation is fundamental to autonomy, health, well-being and justice.
3. Occupational science generates knowledge about the rich diversity of human occupation and about cultural, political, financial and other conditions needed to support meaningful occupation for individuals and communities in diverse world contexts.
4. Occupational science embraces a multidisciplinary, multiperspective approach to research, debate and activism.

ISOS has four main aims:

1. To promote study and research of humans as occupational beings, within the context of their communities and overall society, and the organization of occupation in society.
2. To disseminate information to increase a general understanding of people's occupational needs and the contribution of occupation to the health and well-being of communities.
3. To advocate for occupational justice internationally.
4. To encourage a range of disciplines to consider and frame their own research from an occupational perspective so they may expand their influence on social, political, environmental and occupational processes.

and structure, operating as separate bodies, yet interacting with and supporting each other.

The next task for the ISOS working party was the development of its mission statement (see Table 12.1). The archives reveal that the statement was generated over time from a series of lengthy telephone calls and emails between working party members.[1] It was disseminated to ISOS members for approval on 30 June 2000 and accepted by 5 July 2000.

This bold agenda certainly reflects the dialogue on occupational justice that was initiated by Wilcock and Townsend (2000) at the 1999 conference workshop in which the working party members engaged. The focus on occupational justice, which has remained as a core focus of ISOS for a decade, is what differentiates ISOS from the national occupational science groups that have primarily concentrated on education and dissemination of occupational science research.

[1] The members of the working party which developed the proposal for an international occupational science society and submitted it to WFOT were: H. Barrett, L. do Rozario, M. Molineux, L. Oke, E. Townsend, G. Whiteford, A. Wicks, A. Wilcock and V. Wright-St Clair.

With the vision and mission statement complete, an executive body was then required to implement a strategic plan. Nominees for the inaugural ISOS Board were sought from the founding members of the society and those interested and involved in occupational science. In December 2000, Ann Wilcock was elected President and Elizabeth Townsend and Florence Clark were elected as Vice Presidents. I was recruited as Executive Assistant to coordinate the activities to achieve the ISOS aims. The first task was to establish an electronic listserv to facilitate communication between its members. A website was later developed for electronic dissemination of information about the new discipline of occupational science and to raise awareness of the existence of ISOS. These virtual activities paved the way for a series of face-to-face meetings of occupational scientists from various countries to discuss future directions, and educational workshops open to people interested in learning more about the potential of occupational science.

The first real meeting convened by ISOS was the Inaugural International Occupational Science Think Tank, hosted by the Australasian Occupational Science Centre in Nowra, Australia in July 2006. The think tank delivered on the ISOS mission by bringing together high-profile occupational science researchers and academics from around the world to meet each other for the first time, form networks and begin the debate on the way forward for ISOS. This event certainly stimulated enthusiasm for supporting the international growth of occupational science, and another international think tank was considered essential to maintain the momentum. The second think tank convened by ISOS was held in April 2007, on Catalina Island, off the south coast of California, USA and hosted by USC's Division of Occupational Science and Occupational Therapy. The main objective of this think tank was to implement processes for utilizing this renewed energy for further developing ISOS and occupational science. Subsequently, ISOS hosted an educational workshop in collaboration with ENOTHE in Berlin in 2008, and two workshops in 2010, one during the WFOT Congress in Santiago and the other at the Joint CSOS–SSO:USA conference in London, Ontario. Whilst in Santiago, ISOS also collaborated with the Chilean Society for the Study of Occupation to host a meeting of 40 invited participants, representing 16 countries.

As this narrative reveals, the ISOS programme of activities has been gradually developing momentum overtime. In the beginning, time and energy were focused on establishing a membership base and a means of networking virtually, but more recently, ISOS has been able to organize and host international meetings and workshops. The intent, structure and implementation of the developing ISOS programme are clearly related to the ideological framework underpinning ISOS.

Ideological frameworks shaping ISOS activities

Although there is no written or recorded account of the philosophical framework structuring ISOS, the key beliefs about occupation and occupational science stated in the 2000 mission statement reveal that ideals about justice, inclusivity and diversity are prominent. Interestingly, but not surprisingly, such ideals have epistemological and ontological synergy with the philosophical foundations of occupational science, as espoused by its founders (Wilcock, 1993; Wilcock & Townsend, 2000; Yerxa, 1989).

Advocating occupational justice

Since it was established and throughout its development, ISOS has advocated occupational justice, maintaining that all people have the right to opportunities to develop occupational skills and be engaged in occupations from which they can derive not only subsistence and well-being but a sense of self, purpose and accomplishment. Occupational justice combines two sets of complex ideas (Wilcock & Townsend, 2000); an occupational perspective, derived from the theory of the human as an occupational being (Wilcock, 1993) and ideas about human equity related to the United Nation's Universal Declaration of Human Rights (UN, 1948). The WFOT Position Statement on Human Rights (2006) synthesizes these two concepts of occupation and human rights in the following principles:

- People have the right to participate in a range of occupations that enable them to flourish, fulfil their potential and experience satisfaction in a way consistent with their culture and beliefs.
- People have a right to be supported to participate in occupation and through engaging in occupation to be included and valued as members of their family, community and society.
- The right to occupation encompasses civic, educative, productive, social, creative, spiritual and restorative occupations. The expression of the human right to occupation will take different forms in different places, because occupations are shaped by their cultural, societal and geographic context.

ISOS has directly and indirectly influenced WFOT in accepting the radical ideas in this position statement. First, the statement was developed by the International Advisory Group: Human Rights, a product of the ISOS proposal to establish international advisory groups. And second, the IAG:OS had already sensitized WFOT to this way of thinking by its definitions of occupational therapy (WFOT, 2004), and occupational justice[2] and its position statement on occupational science (WFOT, 2010). These documents, accepted by the WFOT council, emphasize occupation as both the means and the end in occupational therapy, and recognize engagement in occupation as both a human need and a human right.

Being committed to inclusiveness, diversity and dialogue

The second ideological framework that influences the ISOS programme is related to a commitment to inclusiveness and diversity as a way of creating an organization in which all those interested in occupation can engage in dialogue with people around

[2] Occupational justice expands on the concept of social justice which overlooks injustices related to participation in daily life occupations – injustices related to doing rather than having. The concept of occupational justice recognizes that equality or sameness can produce injustices because of human and social and occupational differences (submitted to WFOT by IAG:OS in June 2005).

the world. This commitment relates directly to the fourth belief in the 2000 ISOS Mission Statement: 'Occupational science embraces a multidisciplinary, multiperspective approach to research, debate and activism'. Moreover, ISOS celebrates the diverse ways in which occupational science is developing around the world and supports the belief that contributions from scholars from diverse geographical and cultural locations will expand how occupation is conceptualized and studied (Laliberte Rudman *et al.*, 2008). Such diversity results from the varying degrees to which the science is coupled with practice, the different interests and skills of researchers undertaking occupational science research, the extent of collaboration with and support from other disciplines, and the epistemologies and ontologies underpinning occupational science research and education programmes. As a way of ensuring inclusiveness, ISOS has always invited any self-professed occupational scientist and all individuals and institutions interested in the study of occupation to become members. Membership is open to people from all countries with different philosophical, academic and professional backgrounds.

A survey conducted by ISOS in 2008, to which 32% of the members at that time responded, provides evidence that its membership is geographically and academically diverse. As Table 12.2 shows, in June 2008 the responding members, who identified as managers, researchers, clinicians and educators, resided in 18 different countries. The survey also revealed the various disciplines of those members with doctoral degrees: nursing studies, education, sociology, health science, medical science, anthropology, epidemiology, public health science, health and rehabilitation science, educational

Table 12.2 Country of residence of ISOS membership survey respondents in June 2008

	Country of residence	No. of ISOS members
1	Australia	14
2	Canada	12
3	Denmark	1
4	England	15
5	Germany	1
6	Greece	1
7	Ireland	8
8	Japan	6
9	New Zealand	3
10	Norway	1
11	Portugal	1
12	Scotland	1
13	South Africa	4
14	Sweden	1
15	Taiwan	2
16	United States	13
17	Wales	2
18	The Netherlands	1
		TOTAL 87

psychology, management health and social care. Such diverse disciplinary backgrounds create opportunities for interdisciplinary and intercultural dialogue.

The idea of intercultural dialogue takes as its starting point the recognition of difference and multiplicity of the world in which we live, acknowledging that differences of opinion, viewpoints and values exist not only within each culture but also between cultures. Dialogue in this instance refers to enriching interaction which encourages the respectful sharing of ideas and an exploration of the different thought processes through which the world is perceived and understood (IAU, 2010). Associated with effective dialogue are mutual respect and critical thinking, which are both required and fostered through the dialogic processes (Freire, 1975). ISOS recognizes that intercultural dialogue is a very effective means of gathering and disseminating a diverse range of ideas about occupation and occupational science as well as promoting development of broader self-knowledge and world views (IAU, 2010). In order for ISOS to enable dialogue to occur, it needs to ensure there are opportunities for participation in dialogue.

Adopting participatory approaches

The participatory approaches adopted by ISOS relate to the third ideological framework governing the way ISOS operates in its virtual world. The essence of participatory approaches is the provision of sufficient structure to facilitate discussion in addition to having an open process to allow discussion to find its own course (Carson & Hart, 2005). To enable discussion via electronic participation, the Occupational Science listserv was established in 2001, and a member website with access to discussion fora was set up in 2007. Despite a growing number of registered members and the current popularity worldwide of electronic social networking, the electronic interaction among members was disappointingly low for several years. The introduction of more user-friendly ISOS Google groups in 2010 and the subsequent opportunity to participate in a facilitated online discussion resulted in an energetic and stimulating discussion among members from all around the world.

Members have opportunity to participate electronically in making decisions about ISOS. For example, all members were invited in September 2008 to vote on two Special Resolutions: one resolution was to change the number of Executive members from three to five; and the other was to make a minor modification to its name, ensuring people who did not, or could not, call themselves occupational scientists would still be willing to join the society. ISOS now stands for the International Society for Occupational Science. It is envisaged that by engendering a sense of individual ownership, such participatory opportunities may strengthen allegiance to and support for the Society.

Representativeness is also associated with participatory approaches and can facilitate the capturing of voices that are seldom heard (Carson & Hart, 2005). For example, ISOS endeavoured to ensure representativeness at the first and second think tanks by balancing the invitation list across research agendas, geographical regions, and involvement in education, publication, leadership, scholarship and practice founded on occupational justice. At the first think tank, the 19 participants represented 9 countries,

6 occupational science-related groups and the *Journal of Occupational Science*. In addition, two participants who were not associated directly with academic institutions, but rather work in the field, were invited to represent unheard voices in the communities in which they serve. The 27 participants from 14 countries who attended the second think tank represented 10 different occupational science groups and organizations. Both Brazil and Chile were represented at the second think tank, ensuring the South American voice was audible, joining representatives from the Americas, Asia-Pacific, Africa and Europe.

These three interrelated ideological frameworks shape ISOS activities, albeit implicitly rather than explicitly. The underlying philosophies and basic beliefs are clearly embedded within statements produced by ISOS and are apparent in the programmes it develops. Consequently, the contributions made by ISOS to the development of occupational science reflect these ideologies.

ISOS contributions to the development of occupational science

In terms of contributions to the development of occupational science, ISOS is primarily a facilitator. For the past 10 years, through electronic communications, workshops and think tanks, it has been enabling international collaborations in research and education and promoting intercultural dialogue about the future directions of occupational science. In addition, through printed and electronic publications, it has been sharing with the global occupational science community outcomes of some of the dialogical processes it has facilitated. For example, Occupational Science: Generating an International Perspective (Wicks, 2006) is the report on the Inaugural International Occupational Science Think Tank. The report describes the think tank objectives, summarizes the processes and details the outcomes of the discussions among the participants. An electronic copy of the report is freely available, enabling its wide dissemination with the intent of promoting critical thinking about the development of the science. The vision for occupational science that the think tank participants developed is the core of this report. It reads:

> *In 2016, occupational science will be a cohesive, dynamic and diverse science which transforms practice, is mainstream, is socially and ecologically responsible with innovative partnerships, and which is socially and politically influential.* (Wicks, 2006, p. 11)

Using this vision as a base, the participants then developed ideas on how this vision could be realized. These suggestions, reproduced in Box 12.1, formed a proposal for strategic directions which the participants gifted to the occupational science community.

An example of how this report has stimulated critical thinking is the article published by a group of six Canadian doctoral students and their supervisor (Laliberte Rudman *et al.*, 2008). The think tank vision served as a starting point for their discussions and reflections on the disciplinary culture of occupational science. As an outcome of their deliberations, they shared their vision for occupational science, addressed issues

Box 12.1 Strategic directions to facilitate the development of occupational science, developed by think tank participants, 2006 (Wicks, 2006)

- Continuation of think tanks as a way of building on the TT2006 vision and promoting further dialogue and action related to occupational science
- Development of a pluralistic science
- Development of ISOS as an international organization to support the growth of occupational science internationally
- Development of structures and processes to facilitate theoretical and empirical work regarding occupation – locally, nationally and internationally
- Further dialogue regarding the relationship of occupational science to various types of partners, especially occupational therapy
- Further dialogue regarding the role of occupational science in relation to knowledge development, knowledge dissemination and translation, and social action
- Strategic positioning of occupational science in the mainstream via a focus on targeted areas of social and political relevance.

relating to the identity of occupational science and its relationship to practice, and queried whether occupational science should be interdisciplinary and international.

The Way Forward Plan (Asaba *et al.*, 2007) is another example of an ISOS-generated product intended to influence the future directions of occupational science. This operational and strategic plan was developed by an interim ISOS executive elected at the second think tank. Via emailing and teleconferencing, the five members of the interim executive, representing Australasia, Europe, Asia, North and South America, refined the key functions of ISOS to ensure they were achievable and realistic within its resource constraints. The interim executive also identified areas on which ISOS should focus to facilitate the development of occupational science. The final plan was a comprehensive five-year programme of strategies and activities to achieve its aims and address its focus areas. This plan, a summary of which is provided in Table 12.3, is also available on the ISOS website for individuals and institutions seeking ways to collaborate in research and/or in education programmes.

Since October 2007, when the interim executive was elected to serve a three-year term as the second ISOS Board, some of the activities suggested in the Plan have been either implemented or supported by ISOS. For example, the ISOS website has been gradually upgraded, providing links to relevant websites and organizations, improving electronic communication options for members and offering Spanish, Chinese and Japanese translations of its content; a database of relevant journal articles has been developed for members; workshops on occupational science have been conducted in Berlin, in Santiago, Chile and in London, Canada; newsletters with updates on important issues and events related to occupational science have been disseminated to ISOS members; and ISOS has supported the Occupational Justice Symposium and Think Tank, hosted by the University of Cape Town in 2009. Whilst acknowledging these achievements, there is potential for much more to be done. Addressing some of the challenges facing ISOS will increase its productivity.

Table 12.3 *The Way Forward Plan* 2007–2012 (Asaba *et al.*, 2007)

Aims	Strategies	Activities
1. To facilitate international collaboration in research on occupation Focus areas: • A broad range of approaches to knowledge generation • Cross-cultural research • Mentoring and support of doctoral level research students • Scholar exchange	**1.1.** Establishing an online community of occupation-based researchers	General listserv for members Research Interest Group listservs Message board Discussion board Calendar of occupational science and other relevant symposia and conferences Links to relevant symposia and conferences Databases of past, present and proposed occupation-based research – categorized by topic, context, methods, etc. Database of occupational science research literature – link to JOS Database of members' research interests and expertise Positions vacant/wanted – postings re doctoral and post-doctoral research opportunities or requests
	1.2. Supporting and collaborating with national occupational science and other relevant groups to organize research workshops	ISOS-supported workshops at ENOTHE and WFOT congresses ISOS support of programmes organized by national occupational science groups, e.g. think tanks, doing tanks, symposia
	1.3. Supporting doctoral student research	Travel grants/stipends to students Speaker awards Billeting of students at symposia etc.

(*continued*)

Table 12.3 (*Continued*)

Aims	Strategies	Activities
2. To facilitate international collaboration in the development and delivery of occupational science/occupation-based curricula at all levels of education Focus areas: • A broad range of approaches to knowledge generation • Cross-cultural research • Mentoring and support of doctoral level research students • Scholar exchange	**2.1.** Establishing an online community of occupation-based educators	General listserv for members Message board Discussion board Education Interest Group listserv Links to occupational science/ occupation-based educational programmes Calendar of occupational science and relevant symposia and conferences Database of members' education interests/expertise Positions vacant/wanted – postings of educator and post-grad. teaching opportunities or requests Database + reviews of relevant texts, books and films
3. To promote occupation for health and community development in policy and practice arenas at local, national and international levels Focus areas: • Occupational perspective of health • Transference of evidence to practice • Translation of knowledge to policy	**3.1.** Increasing awareness of occupation and occupational science among the general public, government officers and academics	Publication of occupation-based stories in mainstream media Letters to the Editors Position papers Members' publication of occupation-based research in high-impact scholarly journals Members' presentations of occupation-focused papers at various symposia/ conferences Members' participation in interdisciplinary research, education programmes and conferences

		Support and promotion of occupation-focused continuing professional development programmes
	3.2. Supporting partners and relevant associations	Continued support for and collaboration with JOS and ENOTHE Support of national occupational science organizations
	3.3. Joining relevant organizations, e.g. WHO, UN	Responses to issues re social, economic and community development.

Challenges facing ISOS

The challenges that ISOS faces in relation to achieving its objectives stem primarily from its limited resources. The national occupational science societies face similar challenges. At this point in time, especially when compared to the traditional sciences, occupational science is new, relatively unknown, with a small number of proponents who are scattered around the world. Consequently, there is a small pool from which to draw people who are willing to take on active roles in the development of networks and the promotion of the science. Additionally, as ISOS does not yet have a financial base to cover the cost of paid administrators, it is reliant on a small number of individuals and institutions who volunteer their services. As is the usual case, the volunteers have professional and academic commitments and sometimes have difficulty including ISOS activities into their already busy schedules.

Limited financial resources create other important hurdles for ISOS. For example, ISOS cannot afford for the executive members to meet face to face on a regular basis, so they use email for correspondence and Skype for teleconferences, thereby keeping the directs costs for administrative tasks to nil. Whilst cost-effective, however, electronic meetings and communications are less efficient than face-to-face meetings. Financial constraints also hinder the development of the ISOS website as the major means of communication with the general public, other disciplines and members. A website manager is an essential member of the team to ensure the site is regularly updated and maintained. However, few current members are willing or have the necessary web maintenance skills to take on the role of web manager and ISOS is unable to pay for one.

Sourcing a sustainable revenue base would alleviate these challenges. In 2008, ISOS invited institutions around the world to subscribe to ISOS as institutional members by payment of a moderate fee using an electronic banking transfer. Their subscriptions are one source of revenue for ISOS, and in return for their financial support the institutions receive the newsletters and are acknowledged on the website. While seven institutions subscribed as members, it became apparent that alternative forms of payment were required. A Paypal facility has since been added to the website in the hope that additional institutions may become subscribers. It has also become apparent that many institutions face budgetary constraints themselves, do not have discretionary funds available and could have difficulty explaining the benefits of subscribing to a virtual society. The outcome of an invitation made to individual ISOS members early in 2010 to re-register via the new website where they can join Google discussion groups, and make a donation, if they choose, to assist in the costs associated with administration, was awaited with anticipation. The ISOS Board acknowledges that individuals also have personal budgets to balance and competing professional interests and some individuals may already have subscribed to national occupational science societies. For these reasons, the Board decided not to specify an amount payable by members, and instead, has given members the option of making a donation of any amount. By October 2010, the number of registered members was 175 and the number of donations received was four. Website data shows that spikes in the number of registrants was directly related to the workshops and the facilitated discussion. Such data is useful for planning future programmes for potential and current members.

From a practical perspective, the very principles and beliefs that ISOS upholds as critical for its membership, such as diversity and inclusiveness, create challenges related to communication with and dissemination of information to its members. As a consequence of being open to anyone, in any country, who is interested in occupational science, ISOS members are a very diverse group. Differences in languages, varying access to technology, different levels of understanding and conceptualizations of the science, and even the different time zones of the countries in which members live make it difficult for ISOS to communicate with members in a manner it considers equitable. For example, due to the different time zones in which the current ISOS Board reside, their teleconferences start at 6.00 a.m. for one member, while it is 11.00 p.m. for another. Certainly, the provision of Spanish, Chinese and Japanese translations on the website is addressing the language differences, at least for some members. Setting up such member services requires commitment from members with the requisite skills. Yet despite these challenges and limitations, ISOS has been successful in gradually increasing the number and strength of international networks among occupational scientists and promoting the science through its education programmes and dissemination of information.

Proposals for a sustainable ISOS

As a virtual society with limited resources, ISOS can nonetheless strive to be an effective facilitator of the international development of occupational science. As the only international organization supporting occupational science, it plays a crucial role in establishing and maintaining links with individual occupational scientists and institutions around the world. Hence, all proposals for its sustainability warrant consideration because only a sustainable and viable society can be an effective collective voice advocating occupational justice.

In view of the challenges that ISOS faces and as these are similar to the challenges faced by the national groups, a federation comprised of all the national groups with ISOS as the hub is a possible solution. There are several reasons the federation model is considered appropriate: that model is ideal for combining partners of all shapes and sizes and ownership patterns into a coherent whole; it allows independent units to collaborate without losing their own identity; no one body can dictate to the rest; and, it is both centralist and decentralist, that is, it keeps to the centre those functions and decisions that can most usefully be done there, while allowing everything else to be carried out by the parts (Handy, 2002). The proposal for creating a federation of occupational science societies could engender savings for each society, as some of the common tasks could be streamlined and associated costs would be shared. The economies of scale as well as the resultant synergies when like-minded organizations work collaboratively and share resources would produce benefits for all members of the federation. Additionally, rather than having its own membership and seeking donations, the national societies could be the members of ISOS and an equitable premium, payable to ISOS by each society could be negotiated. But most importantly, if the proposal for an occupational science federation was adopted, ISOS could then focus on its primary role of facilitation, serve as the common link for all the societies and be the international voice of occupational science.

While the formation of a federation may be a long-term solution for the sustainability of ISOS, some short-term strategies need consideration as well. For example, finding an institution that is willing to give ISOS a 'home' could be a means of ensuring that the website is maintained regularly and professionally by website experts. As the website is really the crux of its efforts to facilitate networking, this proposal is certainly worth investigating. Raising awareness of occupational science among professionals other than occupational therapists would also help in promoting the science. Individual occupational scientists could contribute to the awareness-raising by presenting their research at conferences attended by people from various disciplines and seeking publication in a broad range of journals that share the ISOS concern for health, well-being and justice. Both networking and promotion will add to the bank of occupational science champions, who have been the essential factor in keeping ISOS alive thus far, and will be necessary to further the contribution of ISOS to the occupational science community.

Understanding and meeting the needs of members and stakeholders are also requirements for sustainability. Hence, ISOS needs to explore ways of ensuring the channels of communication it provides are effective. Given that social networking by virtual means is so popular worldwide, it is somewhat surprising that the uptake of the interactive fora available through the ISOS website has been slow. Comments from a young student participant at the workshop in London, Ontario suggested that perhaps ISOS could explore setting up a Facebook as a means of encouraging more interaction. Perhaps creating separate educational, research and practice programmes within ISOS, essentially segmenting the ISOS membership, may help to target specific needs and stimulate electronic discussions. For example, occupational science educators may wish to talk with other educators about their need for current, cutting-edge text books, while a forum for researchers could share ideas about funding sources and ways of facilitating multisite research. Collectively, practitioners from around the world could develop strategies for translating evidence from occupational science research into practice. Taking lessons from ENOTHE, which has been very successful in creating interaction and transcending national and cultural borders, is another suggestion which could enable ISOS to develop the ways and means of implementing the range of activities that have been identified in *The Way Forward Plan* (Asaba *et al.*, 2007).

Conclusion

The contribution ISOS has made over the last 10 years to the international development of occupational science through facilitation of networks and intercultural dialogue has been important, albeit subliminal at times. Thus far, with its focus on inclusivity, ISOS has made links with groups and people who previously would have been excluded from opportunities to understand the potential of occupational science. By providing virtual and real forums for dialogue, it has developed international perspectives on the way forward for occupational science.

As someone who has been closely involved in ISOS over the past 10 years, I personally feel the outcomes in relation to occupational justice advocacy have been too few and the development of international networks, too slow. Outsiders may disagree, especially those who had not previously been aware of ISOS. Regardless, the grand vision of creating a worldwide network of occupational scientists advocating occupational justice for health and well-being has yet to be realized. So there are some critical issues that still need to be addressed and practical solutions are required to overcome the challenges that ISOS faces.

Strategies are necessary to effectively engage diverse individuals, in different parts of the world, with their own understandings of occupational science in such a way that ISOS remains inclusive. At the same time, the suggestion to harness the collective strength of the national societies by forming a federation with ISOS at the hub is worthy of consideration. Perhaps the federation could become the international voice representing occupational science, while the national groups focus on addressing the needs of their own members within their own countries. One thing that seems certain is that ISOS will survive and continue evolve, as long as it is energized by a group of people sharing a common passion. It is the passion for occupational justice that is the critical resource for ISOS.

References

Asaba, E., Blanche, E., Jonsson, H., Laliberte Rudman, D., & Wicks, A. (2007). *The Way Forward Plan*. ISOS Interim Executive. Retrieved from http://ahsri.uow.edu.au/content/groups/public/@web/@chsd/@aosc/documents/doc/uow094139.pdf (last accessed 30 June 2011).

Canadian Society of Occupational Scientists (CSOS). (2010). *CSOS mission*. Retrieved from www.csoscanada.com/

Carson, L., & Hart, P. (2005). What randomness and deliberation can do for community engagement. Peer reviewed paper presented at the *International Conference on Engaging Communities*, 14–17 August, Brisbane, Australia. Retrieved from http://www.engagingcommunities2005.org/abstracts/Carson-Lyn-final.pdf (last accessed 3 July 2011).

Clark, F., & Lawlor, M. (2009). The making and mattering of occupational science. In E.B. Crepeau, E.S. Crohn, & B.A.B. Schell (Eds), *Willard and Spackman's Occupational Therapy* (11th ed., pp. 2–24). Philadelphia: Lippincott, Williams & Wilkins.

Dickie, V., Cutchin, M., & Humphry, R. (2006). Occupation as a transactional experience: A critique of individualism in occupational science. *Journal of Occupational Science*, **13**, 83–93.

Freire, P. (1975). *Pedagogy of the Oppressed*. Harmondsworth: Penguin.

Glover, J. (2009). The literature of occupational science: A systematic, quantitative examination of peer-reviewed publications from 1996-2006. *Journal of Occupational Science*, **16**, 92–103.

Handy, C. (2002). *The Elephant and the Flea*. London: Arrow.

International Association of Universities (IAU). (2010). *What is Intercultural Dialogue?* Retrieved from www.iau-aiu.net/

International Society for Occupational Science (ISOS). (2009). *ISOS History*. Retrieved from www.isoccsci.org/

Kielhofner, G. (1997). *Conceptual Foundations of Occupational Therapy* (2nd ed.) Philadelphia: F.A. Davis.

Laliberte Rudman, D., Dennhardt, S., Fok, D. *et al.* (2008). A vision for occupational science: Reflecting on our disciplinary culture. *Journal of Occupational Science*, **15**, 136–46.

Molineux, M., & Whiteford, G. (2005). Occupational science: Genesis, evolution and future contribution. In E. Duncan (Ed.), *Foundations for Practice in Occupational Therapy* (4th ed., pp. 297–312). Edinburgh: Churchill Livingstone.

Molke, D., Laliberte Rudman, D., & Polatajko, H. (2004). The promise of occupational science: A developmental assessment of an emerging academic discipline. *Canadian Journal of Occupational Therapy*, **71**, 269–80.

Pierce, D., Atler, K., Baltisberger, J. *et al.* (2010). Occupational science: A data-based American perspective. *Journal of Occupational Science*, **16**, 204–15.

Society for the Study of Occupation:USA (SSO:USA). (2005). *SSO:USA Mission*. Retrieved from http://www.sso-usa.org/about.htm (last accessed 26 June 2011).

Whiteford, G., Klomp, N., & Wright-St Clair, V. (2005). Complexity theory: Understanding occupation, practice and context. In G. Whiteford & V. Wright-St Clair (Eds), *Occupation and Practice in Context* (pp. 3–15). Marrickville, Australia: Elsevier.

Whiteford, G., Townsend, E., & Hocking, C. (2000). Reflections on a renaissance of occupation. *Canadian Journal of Occupational Therapy*, **67**, 61–9.

Wicks, A. (2006). *Occupational Science: Generating an International Perspective*. Report on the Inaugural International Occupational Science Think Tank. Shoalhaven Campus, University of Wollongong, July 2006. Retrieved from http://ahsri.uow.edu.au/content/groups/public/@web/@chsd/@aosc/documents/doc/uow094114.pdf (last accessed 30 June 2011).

Wilcock, A. (1991). Occupational science. *British Journal of Occupational Therapy*, **54**, 297–300.

Wilcock, A. (1993). A theory of the human need for occupation. *Journal of Occupational Science: Australia*, **1**, 17–24.

Wilcock, A. (1998). Reflections on doing, being and becoming. *Canadian Journal of Occupational Therapy*, **65**, 248–56.

Wilcock, A., & Townsend, E. (2000). Occupational terminology interactive dialogue: Occupational justice. *Journal of Occupational Science*, **7**, 84–6.

World Federation of Occupational Therapists (WFOT). (2002). *Minimum Standards for the Education of Occupational Therapists*. Perth: Author.

World Federation of Occupational Therapists (WFOT). (2004). *World Federation of Occupational Therapists: Definitions of Occupational Therapy from Member Countries Draft 9 2009–2010*. Retrieved from http://www.wfot.org/office_files/DEFINITIONS%20-%20DRAFT9%202009-2010.pdf (last accessed 26 June 2011).

World Federation of Occupational Therapists (WFOT). (2006). *Position Statement on Human Rights*. Retrieved from http://www.wfot.org/office_files/Human%20Rights

%20Position%20Statement%20Final%20NLH%281%29.pdf (last accessed 26 June 2011).

World Federation of Occupational Therapists (WFOT). (2010). Position paper; Occupational science © CM2006. *WFOT Bulletin, 61*, May, 17.

World Health Organization (WHO). (1986). *Ottawa Charter for Health Promotion (online)*. Canadian Public Health Association. Retrieved from http://www.who.int/hpr/NPH/docs/ottawa_charter_hp.pdf (last accessed 30 June 2011).

United Nations. (1948). *Universal Declaration of Human Rights*. Retrieved from http://www.un.org/en/documents/udhr/ (last accessed 26 June 2011).

Yerxa, E. (1989). Occupational science: A renaissance of service to humankind through knowledge. *Occupational Therapy International*, 7, 87–98.

Part V

Visioning a way forward

13 Occupation, inclusion and participation

Gail E. Whiteford and Robert B. Pereira

Occupational science as a discipline is still comparatively new and though there has been a significant leap forward in terms of conceptual and theoretical development in the last decade, much work still needs to be done. Specifically, occupational science and the community of researchers and scholars that contribute to it internationally need to test the utility of foundational concepts, and those currently emerging, against other discursive constructions. As an essentially human science, it needs to 'read' its constructions and pre-understandings of people relative to those generated in other human sciences. This predicates substantive development and concomitant articulation of concepts and constructs of the human-in-the-world. Specifically, in this chapter, we focus on inclusion and participation as constructs fundamental to the project described in this book.

As may be evident in the chapters presented thus far, the development of a more critical ontology has also been important in foregrounding occupational science as a discipline able to make a cogent contribution to current and future (essentially occupational) global phenomena; the rise of the 'working poor', the growing numbers of dislocated persons worldwide due to conflict or natural disaster, underemployment, and retirement of increasingly ageing populations to name but a few. In order to realize the broader societal contribution that it may make, however, occupational science as a corpus of knowledge requires attention in order to both move it from its current position of relative naïveté and to address inherent epistemological tensions arising from an historically Eurocentric orientation.

Occupational Science: Society, Inclusion, Participation, First Edition.
Edited by Gail Whiteford and Clare Hocking.

In this chapter we discuss both social inclusion and participation broadly and consider multiple perspectives through which they may be understood. Most significantly, we draw upon the philosophical and conceptual work of Sen and Nussbaum, who focus on capability. We then discuss the nexus between occupation, inclusion and participation and explore this as a site worthy of greater scholarly and research attention. To inform the discussion, we present some preliminary data from Pereira's study of poverty and participation, to highlight the need for such work from an experiential perspective. Finally, we close with some reflections on ways in which insights generated through focused research may be disseminated and politicized in order to have maximal impact on everyday practices, capacity building and policy development.

Social inclusion: An evolving discourse

> *...[social inclusion provides] an opportunity to analyse the variety of ways that people may be denied full participation in society and the full rights of citizenship.* (Lister, 1999, p. 2)

Social inclusion can be described as being centrally concerned with people and populations having opportunities to participate in society and to enact their rights of citizenship in everyday life. Attempts to define and essentialize social inclusion outside the socio-political context in which it was originally named and framed are, however, problematic. This is because social inclusion is situated within largely Eurocentric conceptual terrain in which notions of equity, justice and citizenship are underpinned by particular religious, philosophical and political histories. Scholars have, for example, challenged the very linguistic arrangement of the concept, focusing on the selection of the terms 'social' and 'inclusion', which supposedly aim to promote and enable participation (Labonte, 2004). Does the 'social' in social inclusion mean in conjunction with another person or people? Does it mean being a member or citizen in a society or population? Is it individualistic or collective in nature, or a combination of both? With respect to 'inclusion', the majority of its critique focuses on questions such as 'inclusion into what?' (Buckmaster & Thomas, 2009) and 'how can one "include" people and groups into structured systems that have systematically "excluded" them in the first place?' (Labonte, 2004, p. 115).

Gould (2006) described the 'taken-for-granted' nature of social inclusion and suggested that an historical *intuitive presumption* in policy has led to the absence of formal definitions of either social inclusion or social exclusion until recently (e.g. in the United Kingdom). Similarly, it has been argued that social inclusion and social exclusion have 'rhetorical power' (Atkinson *et al.*, as cited in Gould, 2006, p. 83), exemplified in the lack of definition across international social policies. Accordingly, determining the success or failure of social inclusion policy and related initiatives becomes problematic because of such an apparently mercurial framing. This is a phenomenon exacerbated by the reluctance of even the European Union to explicitly define social inclusion, describing it instead relative to poverty and social exclusion (European Commission, 2003; Nelms & Tsingas, 2010). Inclusion and participation has also been described as essentially paternalistic and therefore problematic in theory, policy-making and implementation (Taket *et al.*, 2009).

As may be evident then, definitions and conceptualizations of social inclusion reflect 'considerable disparity ... ambiguity and inconsistency in the use and meaning of the term' (Le Boutillier & Croucher, 2010, p. 136). One of the factors contributing to such disparity may well be the scope, scale and complexity of what social inclusion attempts to address, which is in part what makes it such a contested concept (Morrison, 2010; Smyth, 2010; Taket *et al.*, 2009). An area in which there is some agreement, however, is that social inclusion is most usefully viewed as both process and outcome, a framing that we explore in the next section.

Social inclusion as process and outcome: Key concepts

Perhaps the best way to describe how social inclusion can be understood as both process and outcome is to use the analogy of a game of soccer or football. Players go on a field with the aim of scoring a goal. The 'process' of playing together as a team (using strategy, sharing, communication, planning, decision-making, ability and skill), can lead towards scoring a winning goal (or at least attempting to score a goal). One team member cannot do this alone: she or he needs the team and the preceding process of working together. There are also barriers along the way (e.g., out-skilling an opposition player, getting fouled, or being offside) that must be addressed in order for a successful outcome. And whilst such an analogy is admittedly simplistic, community development research into disadvantaged communities in Australia over the past 40 years has come to a similar conclusion as the football analogy: '... in order for services and infrastructural interventions [process] to be effective in the long run, they must not only be useful in their own right [outcome] but simultaneously serve the end of strengthening the overall community [outcome]' (Vinson, 2009, p. 5).

Indeed, most researchers on social inclusion have agreed upon and supported the idea of social inclusion as being a *process* for a person, group, community, organization or population to 'participate' in their society (e.g., Democratic Dialogue, 1995; Levitas, 1996; Lister, 1998; Lombe & Sherraden, 2008; Morrison, 2010; Nelms & Tsingas, 2010; Saloojee, 2001; Saunders, 2003; Smyth, 2010; Ward, 2009; Whiteford & Townsend, 2011). What is also widely acknowledged, however, is the requirement of supportive resources and infrastructure to enable processes of inclusion to be realized.

Conceptual and operational definitions of social inclusion

As has been suggested earlier in this chapter, social inclusion as a term has been problematized and highly contested internationally. Despite this, numerous authors have sought to develop operational definitions, allowing for key ideas to have greater utility and applicability. This is perhaps best evidenced by the works of Levitas *et al.* (2007) and Taket *et al.* (2009), which provided a thorough account of operational definitions constituting the theory and praxis of social exclusion.

In Australia, the Rudd Government considered the following operational definition of social inclusion: 'Social inclusion means building a nation in which all Australians have the opportunity and support they need to participate fully in the nation's economic and community life, develop their own potential and be treated with dignity and respect' (Department of the Prime Minister and Cabinet, 2009, p. 2).

The Rudd Government also acknowledged that being *socially included* (original emphasis) meant that people had the resources, opportunities and capabilities they needed to 'learn' (participate in education and training); 'work' (participate in employment, unpaid or voluntary work including family and carer responsibilities); 'engage' (connect with people, use local services and participate in local, cultural, civic and recreational activities) and 'have a voice' (influence decisions that affect them) (Australian Social Inclusion Board, 2010; Department of Education, Employment and Workplace Relations, 2009; Department of the Prime Minister and Cabinet, 2009). Interestingly, the Rudd Government's operational definition, which has not changed since Julia Gillard took over as Prime Minister on 24 June 2010, has a stronger focus on the material rather than more discursive aspects (Ward, 2009).

Despite the Rudd Government providing a set of social inclusion principles rather than a more formalized definition, the South Australian Government's social inclusion initiative has formally defined it in its policy as:

> *...the creation of a society where all people feel valued, their differences are respected, and their basic needs – both physical and emotional – are met ... Social inclusion is about participation; it is a method for social justice. It is about increasing opportunities for people, especially the most disadvantaged people, to engage in all aspects of community life.* (Government of South Australia, 2009)

The South Australian social inclusion initiative is considered as a world-leading and innovative one by the World Health Organization's Commission on Social Determinants of Health (WHO, 2008), which described it as valuing 'political recognition and strong commitment to inclusion and health equity' (p. 160). Such an endorsement suggests not just an alignment of core values between organizations, but the importance of framing social inclusion as recognition, in which differences are respected and thus politicized.

As may be evident thus far, the complex, multidimensional nature of social inclusion and its historically interdisciplinary development pose a challenge to any attempt at summarizing its conceptual underpinnings. In the next section we move from definitions to a discussion of key ideas that have informed discussions of social inclusion, drawing from different disciplines including occupational science. Because of its universality, we start here with a discussion of inclusion and human rights.

Social inclusion and human rights

> *Social inclusion is about social cohesion plus, it is about citizenship plus, it is about the removal of barriers plus, it is anti-essentialist plus, it is about rights and responsibilities plus, it is about accommodation of differences plus, it is*

> *about democracy plus, and it is about a new way of thinking about the problems of injustice, inequalities and exclusion ... It is the combination of the various pluses that make the discourse on social inclusion so incredibly exciting.* (Saloojee, 2001)

At the inaugural Australian Government social inclusion conference in January 2010, the then Parliamentary Secretary for Social Inclusion, Senator Ursula Stephens claimed that 'social inclusion goes hand-in-hand with human rights' (2010). Due to the recent introduction of social inclusion policy discourse in Australia, what remains untested, however, is the extent to which the Universal Declaration of Human Rights (UN, 1948) is upheld in such policy, especially the declaration's first, overarching article, that 'all human beings are born free and equal in dignity and rights. They are endowed with reason and conscience and should act towards one another in a spirit of brotherhood'. There is an attendant challenge here though. And that is, despite the Universal Declaration of Human Rights (UN, 1948) being a framework through which social inclusion can be enabled, it is in essence aspirational and requires national governments to mandate and monitor it (Stadnyk, Townsend, & Wilcock, 2010). This requires committed vigilance.

The United Kingdom, some years ago now, adopted a human rights 'plus' model. There, Disability Rights Commissioner, Liz Sayce (2001), developed a definition of social inclusion specifically with a focus on the human rights and advocacy of citizens living with disability. In her definition, Sayce described the virtues of social inclusion as including a combination of rights, social and economic access, opportunities and equality of status. Of note, the definition also explicitly endorses a social model of disability. As many readers will be aware, the social model of disability rejected medicalized, deficit constructions of disability in which people living with disability were seen as 'the problem' (Goggin & Newell, 2005; Layton, 2009; Smith, 2009), focusing instead on inclusion as being about the removal of barriers across individual, physical, attitudinal and systemic levels of society (Kahune & Savulescu, 2009; Layton, 2009; Smith, 2009). Again, as a societal aspiration, removal of such barriers systematically and across sectoral boundaries calls for commitment and vigilance as well as 'joined-up' government services (Australian Social Inclusion Board, 2010).

There are sceptics of such a rights-based orientation to social inclusion, however, who argue that it is too broad in scope and therefore too difficult to operationalize (Renner *et al.*, 2007). The risk of not making overt the relationship between social inclusion and human rights is that the focus can, by default, end up on processes of social exclusion. Clearly, this does not serve all members of society as many people 'do not benefit from mainstream development efforts because of who they are or where they live. In addition to poverty, they face discrimination based on social identity' (Renner *et al.*, 2007). Others have argued that rights are compromised when citizens face entrenched discrimination in particular cultural contexts because of a lack of inter-subjective recognition and a concomitant diminishment of dignity and respect (Honneth, 2001; Morrison, 2010). Whilst dignity and respect are important, however, they cannot be cut free from the right to develop and exercise capabilities regardless of context. This is the focus of the next section.

Capabilities and inclusion

The 'capability approach' was developed and theorized by both economist Amartya Sen and philosopher Martha Nussbaum. Nobel prize laureate Amartya Sen (2000) described poverty as not only a state of deprivation of material necessities (e.g., food, water, income shortage or shelter), but also as a state of deprivation of opportunities through which *capabilities* can be developed. Sen (2000) identified that capability deprivation may be a major determinant of exclusion beyond just the financial and suggested that a lack of income per se is not the sole barrier to the development and realization of potential. Sen (2000) has also related a deprivation of capability development as having significant impacts on well-being, thus rendering it an issue of social justice (Fraser, 1995). Accordingly, Nussbaum (2003) described Sen's approach to capabilities as a 'major contribution to the theory of social justice' (p. 33). It should be noted that the capability approach has also been identified as being influential to many academic disciplines and movements such as economics, development studies, disability studies, political philosophy and egalitarianism (Kuklys & Robeyns, 2005; Sen, 1992; Terzi, 2009).

The basic premise of the theory of capability focuses on life as 'consisting of a set of interrelated "functionings", consisting of beings and doings' (1992, p. 39) such as good health, happiness, participating in community life and enjoying a nutritious diet (Sen, 1992, 1993). 'Capability' is closely related to Sen's concept of functionings and encapsulates 'a set of vectors of functionings [ranging from elementary to more complex functionings in nature; e.g. eating and social integration], reflecting the person's freedom to lead one type of life or another' (p. 40). Self-determination and freedom are described as the outcomes of enacting capabilities (Alexander, 2008; Pettit, 2001; Saunders, 2003; Sen, 1992, 2000).

Doings and beings, a conceptual framing of human existence and activity familiar to occupational scientists, are in and of themselves important to realizing capabilities. This of course contrasts with a more utilitarian perspective (e.g. welfare enables capability) where lives are viewed as being enriched through the provision of goods and services (Sen, 1992). Therefore, a person's capability, according to Sen, is dependent on a variety of factors that determine a person's ability to 'do the things that she would choose to do and has reason to choose to do' (Sen, 2001, p. 55). Again, this is a statement that speaks to the close nexus between the concerns of occupational science and the capability approach. This is true also of another key tenet of Sen's work; that of capability deprivation. Consider here the shared concerns of the impacts of deprivation from occupation (Whiteford, 2000; Wilcock, 2006) and Sen's (2000) description of capability deprivation, an idea shaped by Aristotelian thought:

> *The Aristotelian account of the richness of human life was explicitly linked to the necessity to "first ascertain the function of man," followed by exploring "life in the sense of activity." In this Aristotelian perspective, an impoverished life is one without the freedom to undertake important activities that a person has reason to choose.* (pp. 3–4)

Nussbaum has also drawn on Aristotelian philosophy, drawing upon the concept of a 'flourishing human life' as central to understanding different capabilities (Alexander, 2008). These include capabilities that range from having good health and shelter, through to being able to exercise the imagination and being able to laugh, through to being able to participate politically (Nussbaum, 2003). Whilst we do not have the space for an exhaustive discussion of Nussbaum's work here, it is important to note that whilst she and Sen have been key to the development of the capability approach and its contribution to understandings of inclusion, there is a significant point of departure between them (Alexander, 2008; Nussbaum, 2003; Nussbaum as cited in Alexander, 2008; Sen, 2004). Essentially, whilst Sen promoted an open approach to 'advocating a capabilities-based understanding of justice ... without endorsing a definite list of capabilities' (Alexander, 2008, p. 63), Nussbaum described and delineated her exhaustive list of capabilities. This, she felt, was requisite to political action and suggested that Sen had stopped short of this more radical position. Instead she stressed that functionings can actually be assessed and that this might serve as a basis through which inequities could be addressed (Nussbaum, as cited in Alexander, 2008).

So far in this chapter we have presented and discussed concepts central to the development of social inclusion and definitional constructions. Where possible we have also sought to draw the links through to core concerns and foci of occupational science. In order to capture some of these ideas, see Table 13.1 for an overview of what has been discussed thus far. It also introduces some new concepts such as connectedness and solidarity which serve as a useful theoretical resource for the reader in understanding the scope of social inclusion as a guiding idea across many disciplines in the preceding three decades.

In the next section we discuss more explicitly the relationship between social inclusion and occupational science through an examination of participation as inclusion might mean and its relationship to concepts of enablement and empowerment.

Participation: Enablement and empowerment

What is evident across not just the occupational science but social science literature is that it is the doings (or occupations) of individuals and groups in society that are the vehicle through which participation and ultimately inclusion can be achieved. As Miller Polgar and Landry (2004) have suggested, it is not sufficient to understand that a person or community does something per se. Participation encompasses and 'explores what they are doing, why they are doing it, and what it brings to their lives, individually or collectively' (Miller Polgar & Landry, 2004, p. 198).

Of course understanding everyday occupation as participation, and ultimately as inclusion in society, stimulates numerous related questions: for example, what differentiates participation and inclusion? That question begs consideration of the case of Rick Hoyt. Cited in Polatajko *et al.* (2007), this young man with cerebral palsy was pushed by his father as they competed in marathons and triathlons. Was he participating, though not actually running himself? Was he fully engaged? Most certainly,

Key elements	Key concepts/constructs	Key authors
Social inclusion as *capability*	• The basic premise of the capabilities approach focuses on life 'consisting of a set of interrelated "functionings", consisting of beings and doings' (1992, p. 39) such as good health, happiness, participating in community life and enjoying a nutritious diet (Sen, 1992, 1993) • Functionings are constitutive of well-being • 'Capability' is closely related to Sen's concept of functionings and encapsulates 'a set of vectors of functionings [ranging from elementary to more complex functionings in nature; e.g. eating and social integration], reflecting the person's freedom to lead one type of life or another' (1992, p. 40) • Benefits (or outcomes) can include self-determination and freedom to choose the life that one wants through enacting capabilities by achieving sets of functionings • A person's capability is dependent on a variety of factors which determine a person's ability to 'do the things that she would choose to do and has reason to choose to do' (Sen, 2001, p. 55)	Alexander (2008, 2010) Burchardt (2004) Claassen (2009) Nevile (2007) Nussbaum (2003) Sen (1992, 1993, 1999, 2000, 2001, 2004) Sen & Nussbaum (1993) Terzi (2009)
Social inclusion as *opportunity*	• Broader environments and contexts facilitate or provide opportunities • Opportunities enable individuals to use their capabilities and resources to participate as they choose • Self-determination and choice • There is a nexus between capabilities, opportunities and resources for social inclusion (Dept. of Education, Employment and Workplace Relations, 2009; Levitas *et al.*, 2007)	Australian Social Inclusion Board (2010) Dept. of Education, Employment and Workplace Relations (2009) Dept. of the Prime Minister and Cabinet (2010) Levitas *et al.* (2007) Nelms & Tsingas (2010) Sayce (2001) Sen (1999)

Social inclusion as *solidarity*	• Social bonds between the individual and society • Living together peacefully and constructively • Shared system of interdependence • Relationships can be based on cooperation • Contributing to the common good • Capacity of people to come together, despite their differences, in ways that are mutually beneficial (Vasta, 2010a) • 'Valuing forms of life characterized by many social differences' (Bach, 2005, p. 128) • Reciprocity provides a foundation for the realization of rights in relation to others (Bach, 2005)	Bach (2005) Heidegren (2002) Honneth (2001) Saloojee (2001, 2005, 2011) Vasta (2010a, 2010b, 2011)
Social inclusion as *recognition*	• Acknowledges the recognition, acceptance, dignity and respect of a person's or societal group's difference and diversity (Honneth, 2001; Morrison, 2010) • Recognition is reciprocal, incorporating reciprocal respect • Recognition promotes self-respect as a product of an inclusive transaction between individuals or groups that takes place in moral and practical terms (Honneth, 2001) • Personal integrity • Recognizing one another as equal is a moral imperative, rather than being an exclusive human rights imperative • Recognition allows one to value diverse forms of knowledge • Recognition is central to realizing human dignity and equality of worth across interpersonal, institutional and societal levels (Bach, 2005)	Bach (2005) Deranty (2009) Fraser (1995) Heidegren (2002) Honneth (2001) Ikäheimo 2002, 2007, 2009 Ikäheimo & Laitinen (2010) Morrison (2010) Shakespeare (2006)
Social inclusion as *poverty reduction*	• Understanding social inclusion beyond having material goods and services; inclusion is more than market involvement • Considers inclusion through paid employment as limited regarding the realities of other roles, responsibilities and obligations such as care-giving, volunteering and education • Supports poverty as being deprived of 'capabilities'	Fraser (1995, 2000, 2001) Levitas (1996, 1998) Lister 1998, 2004, 2010 Mitchell & Shillington (2005) Morrison (2010) Saunders (2003) Saunders, Naidoo & Griffiths (2007) Sen (2000) Silver (1994)

(*continued*)

Table 13.1 (*Continued*)

Key elements	Key concepts/constructs	Key authors
Social inclusion as *citizenship*	• Key elements of citizenship include having civil rights, political rights and social rights (Kim, 2010) • Realization and enactment of human rights • Freedom to participate and contribute to society • Recognizing the rights, obligations and institutions that play a role in developing and supporting equality of status in the community (Buckmaster & Thomas, 2009, p. 16) • Being a valued citizen • Mutual sharing and upholding equality and respect • Enjoying a basic standard of living	Buckmaster & Thomas (2009) Edwards (2008) Kim (2010) Lister (2010) Saloojee (2001, 2005, 2011) Shergold (2009) Sinclair *et al.* (2007)
Social inclusion as *rights*	• Upholding universal rights and privileges • Celebrating equality, recognition and mutual respect • Rights-based agendas enable harmonious interaction, collaboration and participation • Rights enable participation in cultural, economic, political and social aspects of life • Full participation across social, political and economic processes • Social justice • Potential for active citizen engagement such as being involved in decision-making at the individual, interpersonal, group, organizational, community and societal levels	Edwards (2010) Frazee (2005) Honneth (2001) Government of South Australia (2009) Lombe & Sherraden (2008) Morrison (2010) Nelms and Tsingas (2010) Rawls (1971, 1999) Reiter, (2008) Saloojee, (2001, 2005, 2011) Sayce (2001)
Social inclusion as *means and ends*	• 'Means' for participating in, and contributing to, society • Social inclusion processes enacted by organizations, institutions or governments make them accountable for their actions • Lead to goals or 'outcomes/ends' • Can be measured, evaluated and critiqued for the betterment of society	Democratic Dialogue (1995) Levitas (1996) Lister (1998) Lombe & Sherraden (2008) Morrison (2010) Nelms & Tsingas (2010) Saloojee (2001, 2011) Saunders (2003) Smyth (2008, 2010) Ward (2009) Whiteford & Townsend (2011)

Social inclusion as *connectedness*	• Being actively involved with another person, object, group or environment • Interactions provide and promote comfort and well-being • Sharing bonds and understandings between people which may bring them closer • Culturally relative, e.g. Western perspectives of connectedness (Hagerty *et al.*, 1993; Taket *et al.*, 2009; Townsend & McWhirter, 2005) is epistemologically different to an African perspective of connectedness, or interconnectedness (e.g. *Ubuntu*; Tutu, 1999)	Hagerty *et al.* (1993) Maulana & Eckhardt (2007) Owens (2009) Taket *et al.* (2009) Townsend & McWhirter (2005) Tutu (1999)
Social inclusion as *economic participation*	• Social inclusion through work/employment/productivity • Positive feeling of self-worth through work • Work provides meaning • Economic participation is a means by which people can be integral, productive and contributing members of society	Social Exclusion Task Force (2009) Dept. of the Prime Minister and Cabinet (2009)

from his own accounts. This case prompts us to reconsider just what participation is, especially in an era of increasingly 'virtual' and cyber interactions. For instance, is using Facebook or other social networking sites a form of participation and hence inclusion?

Such questions that examine the inherent complexities of occupational engagement and participation require testing through multiple perspectives and using a range of innovative methodologies. A research agenda focused thus will not only further develop the corpus of knowledge in occupational science (Molineux & Whiteford, 2006) but, when also expanded to understanding what it means to be in forced and oppressive occupations will add significantly to the cross-disciplinary understandings of the 'human condition' (Letts, Rigby, & Stewart, 2003; Miller Polgar & Landry, 2004; Rebeiro, 2001; Strong *et al.*, 1999; Whiteford & Wright-St Clair, 2005). Whilst such focused research needs to be undertaken into the future, however, there have been findings which point to social connectedness as one of the foundational elements of participation. Returning again to the use of social media, it has been found that one of the main enabling factors for participation is having a network of supportive people (Bejerholm, 2010; Pieris & Craik, 2004).

Participation as social inclusion has also been related to the concept of empowerment in both the social and occupational science literature. Empowerment can involve caring for oneself or others, making decisions, advocacy, power sharing, controlling one's circumstances in life and feeling respected, safe, secure, having a sense of belonging as well as having a voice (Luttrell *et al.*, 2009; Shergold, 2009; WHO, 1998). However, a major assumption of the concept of empowerment is that power exists in the first place to either be shared or empower oneself or others (Layton, 2009). As an artefact of the power relations inherent in all nation states, democratically elected or otherwise, some groups enjoy greater power in and control over their everyday lives than others – hence empowerment is relative to context. A corollary of this is the frequent presence of sanctions against types of occupational participation, which further entrenches marginality (Stadnyk *et al.*, 2010). An example of this, at the time of the writing of this book is the case of women in Saudi Arabia. They are unable to vote, travel without written permission, drive or own a bank account (Miller, 2011).

Empowerment from an occupational science perspective is congruent with the concept of enablement. Both are also inherent in an historical view of justice as well as through a conceptual understanding of the theory of recognition (Honneth, 2001), a politics of redistribution (Fraser, 1995; Levitas, 1998; Morrison, 2010) and the capabilities approach (Nussbaum, 2003; Sen, 2000) explored earlier. Extending from such theories, a philosophical view of empowerment and enablement can also be related to Rawls' historical theory of justice (1971) and Young's concept of a 'justice of difference' (1990, as cited in Stadnyk *et al.*, 2010). Empowerment, from Young's 'justice of difference' perspective, highlighted the importance of having 'opportunities' to engage in life. Opportunity, in Young's view, is a concept of 'enablement'; a justice to enable individuals to carry out their occupations and enjoy a life free from exploitation, violence and oppression (Stadnyk *et al.*, 2010). Importantly, the concept of enablement supports the notion of empowerment rather than dependence (Townsend & Brintnell, 1997). In the next section, in which we present narrative data from a study of multiple disadvantages, notions of what constitutes empowerment and how a justice of difference can be problematic in the face of bureaucratic policy are particularly relevant.

Understanding participation and inclusion: Situated research

Having reviewed the theoretical and conceptual terrain of social inclusion and participation, the data presented in this section comes from research focused on citizens living in poverty and with a disability in one of Australia's most socially deprived areas, Western Sydney (Vinson, 2007). Methodologically, the research adopted two distinct approaches: a discourse analysis of the Australian Government's Social Inclusion Policy during the Rudd Labour Government, and a life history approach to understanding the narratives of people living with multiple disadvantages. The purpose of the study overall was to examine the ways in which policy and lived experience 'speak' to each other and in particular highlight points of intersection and/or disjunction. Participants from a range of age and social backgrounds volunteered through two different types of organizations, one an NGO focused on serving the needs of homeless and at-risk individuals and families, the other, a government-funded disability employment service. In recognition of their time, all participants were given a shopping voucher to enable the purchase of food and other essential items. Given that the study was focused on disadvantage and poverty, this was an important recognition of the fact that many lived lives of real and pressing needs.

Whilst we do not have the space to present a comprehensive account of the research and its findings, we present here an extract from one participant's narrative. The participant, whom we have named James, is a 33-year-old single, unemployed man who suffered a work-related injury (and has a resultant disability) 5 years ago. Of note is the fact that he played sport at an elite level and had an agentic orientation to life. We have selected James' narrative as it is a powerful account of the complex interaction between place, identity, social constructions of disability and both federal and state policy, and how this interaction can be experienced as both oppressive and exclusionary.

They lump you in with the losers: Struggling to participate with dignity

> *So, the system at the moment is not ... okay it's good if I wanted to be on the Disability Pension for the rest of my life, and I wanted to live in shared accommodation. And that's what they [The Welfare Agency] are trying to force me to do ... I walk through the shops and people just stare at me like you know, what the hell's wrong with him. It is very uncomfortable, but you get used to it. Um, but to have that normal life, I don't want people looking at me. So it means that I've gotta be able to walk properly. It also means I've got to have my own place. I've got to be able to live strong by myself as a strong individual person. Um, unfortunately, you need income to do that. Unfortunately, I'm stuck between a rock and a hard place it feels like, you know. So, the system really does not help people like me. It only helps people that want to give up and do what the doctors tell them. Which is, sit at home, take it easy, don't do nothing. You know.*

> *... They said that we're not giving any more rent assistance, you're going to have to think about going into shared accommodation. This is where we can put you. I said I don't even want to see that form because I'm not going. I said I am still capable about being in the workforce as a full employee. They said no ... why not? What, because I've got a problem with my leg? You're fat and lazy and you sit behind a desk ... you probably couldn't do the work that I do. That's why you're saying it. But, even [though] I'm disabled, I can still do it. I know I can ... That's just my attitude, you know. Any athlete will tell you that ... all these other people, don't see it that way yeah ... It's a bit nasty and a bit disheartening like I said.*

> *... It's like a dictatorship when you get into the system. They tell you this, this, this and you've got to abide by it. But not everyone's the same, are they? ... And I think that's the problem. They don't take us case by case. They take us as ... and I don't mean this in the worst way ... actually I can say this 'cause I've lived in Western Sydney pretty much all my life. They treat me like another bum, loser that just wants to be on the Disability Pension ... I'm not getting lumped in with all these losers. And that's just the way I like it. You know, but then they 'do' lump you in with the losers when they are looking at you instead of doing the case to case. They just put you in with the losers and say well you've got the same attitude as anyone else in this area. No, I just live in this area because this is all that I can afford. If I had the money, I'd be living closer to the city or something you know. Um, but I just don't like that situation being lumped in with everyone else and categorized. It's just not right. It's not fair and I've been saying it for ages. Something needs to be done about it ... Instead of just saying, this is what everyone will do, you know. 'Cause we are not all the same.*

Discussion

As is evident, the narrative extract presented above is dense and multilayered. In particular, it speaks to the struggles of one man to assert his own identity and enact his capabilities on his own terms. Through the definitions and constraints of being made 'other', that is, as disabled, he describes feeling excluded from opportunities for inclusion through participation.

To what extent does his narrative speak to the earlier conceptual and theoretical framing of inclusion presented in this chapter? First and foremost, the salience of the concept of the capability framework is clearly evident (Burchardt, 2004; Nussbaum, 2003; Sen, 1992, 1993, 1999, 2000; Sen & Nussbaum, 1993). This is a person who has not had opportunities through which to exercise his capabilities. No one has focused on his capabilities and in this respect it seems that the policy represents the antithesis of a capability development ethos. Such a reductionist approach (Saloojee, 2011) from James' account, does not allow him to construct his identity on his own terms. He becomes, as he says, a 'loser', lumped in. The tragedy of such a framing, where capabilities are neither recognized nor enabled, is the experience of being stuck and frustrated; in other words, what James describes as feeling *boxed in*. As Saloojee (2011) suggested, demanding that people conform to a homogenous identity, and a predetermined pathway to 'do' in society, has a significant human cost.

Considered through the lens of James' experience then, consideration of social inclusion as recognition and a human right, also becomes challenging. James describes his experience of failing to be recognized (Honneth, 2001) for who he was, currently is and what he is capable of doing as a potentially productive citizen in society. The question is begged then, to what extent is human potentiality wasted when we deny people the right of valued recognition (Saloojee, 2005). From a rights-based discursive construction of a social inclusion perspective (Lombe & Sherraden, 2008), James' account is also disturbing and causes us to ask, does he have a right to live as he chooses and assert some autonomy in his life? Does he have a right to be self-defining, as not disabled, when being disabled as framed by policy seems to have negative implications for him. The paradox there, of course, is that if he was defined as disabled, he would be in financially better circumstances. The right to assert one's chosen identity, it seems, has an *actual* cost.

Our earlier discussion of social inclusion as means and ends (Lombe & Sherraden, 2008; Morrison, 2010; Saloojee, 2001, 2011; Saunders, 2003; Smyth, 2010; Ward, 2009; Whiteford & Townsend, 2011) is salient here. Denied the means through which he can participate and therefore contribute to society, the 'ends' for James become largely irrelevant. They represent an idealized notion that he cannot relate to. Viewed thus, social inclusion as ends becomes purely aspirational. This is because without the means, the structural vehicles as shaped by policy dictates, inclusion through participation cannot realistically be achieved. In this respect, the nexus with the occupational justice discourse is particularly relevant. In occupational justice, *differences* in capabilities are valued and recognized. Philosophically and conceptually then, occupational justice could have the power to inform policy development in the disability, employment and welfare arenas. Ultimately, this could allow for diverse identities and potentialities to be validated, as James says, case by case, rather than as one homogenous 'lump'.

Conclusions

In this chapter we have presented key ideas that have shaped social inclusion as a discourse internationally. As highlighted throughout, it is a complex and highly contested construct but one which has significant power to inform policy and practice and mobilize resources to those populations most in need. Particular consideration has been devoted here to what constitutes participation, and the intersection between conceptual framings of participation in the international occupational science. We have, as we intended, tested ideational developments from occupational science against those generated in other disciplines and found a strong alignment. It is our opinion that such conceptual alignment could be the basis through which the potential contribution of occupational science could be more fully realized.

Finally, we presented and discussed a narrative from a ground-breaking study into multiple disadvantage read against social inclusion policy in Australia. An analysis of the narrative points to the bald fact that exclusions are experienced everyday by people made marginal due to a complex interweaving of policy, institutional practice and societal practices of 'othering'. Maintaining the balance between holding such experiences up for examination and analysing the discourses that shape them is an ongoing challenge into the future.

References

Alexander, J.M. (2008). *Capabilities and Social Justice: The Political Philosophy of Amartya Sen and Martha Nussbaum*. Aldershot: Ashgate.

Alexander, J.M. (2010). Ending the liberal hegemony: Republican freedom and Amartya Sen's theory of capabilities. *Contemporary Political Theory*, **9**, 5–24.

Australian Social Inclusion Board. (2010). *Social Inclusion in Australia: How Australia is Faring*. Canberra: Department of the Prime Minister and Cabinet.

Bach, M. (2005). Social inclusion as solidarity: Re-thinking the child rights agenda. In T. Richmond & A. Saloojee (Eds), *Social Inclusion: Canadian Perspectives* (pp. 126–54). Toronto: Laidlaw Foundation.

Bejerholm, U. (2010). Relationships between occupational engagement and status of and satisfaction with sociodemographic factors in a group of people with schizophrenia. *Scandinavian Journal of Occupational Therapy*, **17**, 244–54.

Buckmaster, L., & Thomas, M. (2009). *Social Inclusion and Social Citizenship – Towards a Truly Inclusive Society*. Retrieved 24 March 2010, from http://www.aph.gov.au/library/pubs/rp/2009-10/10rp08.pdf

Burchardt, T. (2004). Capabilities and disability: The capabilities framework and the social model of disability. *Disability & Society*, **19**, 735–51. doi: 10.1080/0968759042000284213

Claassen, R.J.G. (2009). New directions for the capability approach: Deliberative democracy and republicanism. *Res Publica: A Journal of Legal and Social Philosophy*, **15**, 421–28. doi: 10.1007/s11158-009-9091-5

Democratic Dialogue. (1995). *Social Exclusion, Social Inclusion: Report No. 2*. Retrieved 23 March 2011, from http://cain.ulst.ac.uk/dd/report2/report2.htm

Department of Education, Employment and Workplace Relations. (2009). *The Australian Public Service social inclusion policy design and delivery toolkit framework*. Canberra: Social Inclusion Unit, Department of the Prime Minister and Cabinet.

Department of the Prime Minister and Cabinet. (2009). *A stronger, fairer Australia: National statement on social inclusion*. Canberra: Department of the Prime Minister and Cabinet.

Deranty, J.-P. (2009). *Beyond Communication: A Critical Study of Axel Honneth's Social Philosophy*. Boston, MA: Brill.

Edwards, K. (2008). Social inclusion and youth participation: A new deal for Australia's young people. *Youth Studies Australia*, **27**, 11–17.

Edwards, K. (2010). Social inclusion: Is this a way forward for young people, and should we go there? *Youth Studies Australia*, **29**, 16–24.

European Commission. (2003). *Communication from the Commission to the Council, the European Parliament, the European Economic and Social Committee and the Committee of the Regions: Joint report on social inclusion summarizing the results of the examination of the National Action Plans for Social Inclusion 2003–2005*. Retrieved 17 February 2010, from http://europa.eu/legislation_summaries/employment_and_social_policy/situation_in_europe/c10616_en.htm

Fraser, N. (1995). From redistribution to recognition? Dilemmas of justice in a 'post-socialist' age. *New Left Review*, **I/212** 68–93.

Fraser, N. (2000). Rethinking recognition. *New Left Review*, **3**, 107–20.
Fraser, N. (2001). Recognition without ethics? *Theory, Culture & Society*, **18**, 21–42. doi: 10.1177/02632760122051760
Frazee, C. (2005). Thumbs up! Inclusion, rights and equality as experienced by youth with disabilities. In T. Richmond & A. Saloojee (Eds), *Social Inclusion: Canadian Perspectives* (pp. 105–25). Toronto: Laidlaw Foundation.
Goggin, G., & Newell, C. (2005). *Disability in Australia*. Sydney: University of New South Wales Press.
Gould, N. (2006). Social inclusion as an agenda for mental health social work: Getting a whole life? *Journal of Policy Practice*, **5**, 77–90.
Government of South Australia. (2009). *People and Community at the Heart of Systems and Bureaucracy: South Australia's social inclusion initiative*. Adelaide: Government of South Australia.
Hagerty, B.M., Lynch-Sauer, J., Patusky, K., & Bouwsema, M. (1993). An emerging theory of human relatedness. *Image – Journal of Nursing Scholarship*, **25**, 291–6.
Heidegren, C-G. (2002). Anthropology, social theory, and politics: Axel Honneth's theory of recognition. *Inquiry*, **45**, 433–6.
Honneth, A. (2001). Recognition or redistribution?: Changing perspectives on the moral order of society. *Theory, Culture & Society*, **18**, 43–55. doi: 10.1177/02632760122051779
Ikäheimo, H. (2002). On the genus and species of recognition. *Inquiry*, **45**, 447–62.
Ikäheimo, H. (2007). Recognizing persons. *Journal of Consciousness Studies: Controversies in Science & the Humanities*, **14**, 224–47.
Ikäheimo, H. (2009). Personhood and the social inclusion of people with disabilities: A recognition-theoretical approach. In K. Kristiansen, S. Vehmas & T. Shakespeare (Eds), *Arguing about Disability: Philosophical Perspectives* (pp. 77–92). Abingdon: Routledge.
Ikäheimo, H., & Laitinen, A. (2010). Esteem for contributions to the common good: The role of personifying attitudes and instrumental value. In M. Seymour (Ed.), *The Plural States of Recognition* (pp. 98–121). Basingstoke: Palgrave Macmillan.
Kahune, G., & Savulescu, J. (2009). The welfarist account of disability. In K. Brownlee & A. Cureton (Eds), *Disability and Disadvantage* (pp. 14–53). Oxford: Oxford University Press.
Kim, H.S. (2010). UN disability rights convention and implications for social work practice. *Australian Social Work*, **63**, 103–16.
Kuklys, W., & Robeyns, I. (2005). Sen's capability approach to welfare economics. In W. Kuklys (Ed.), *Amartya Sen's Capability Approach: Theoretical Insights and Empirical Applications* (pp. 9–30). Berlin: Springer-Verlag.
Labonte, R. (2004). Social inclusion/exclusion: Dancing the dialectic. *Health Promotion International*, **19**, 115–21. doi: 10.1093/heapro/dah112
Layton, K. (2009). Paradoxes and paradigms: How can the social model of disability speak to international humanitarian assistance? *ANU Undergraduate Research Journal*, **1**, 55–61.
Le Boutillier, C., & Croucher, A. (2010). Social inclusion and mental health. *British Journal of Occupational Therapy*, **73**, 136–9. doi: 10.4276/030802210X12682330090578

Letts, L., Rigby, P., & Stewart, D. (Eds). (2003). *Using Environments to Enable Occupational Performance*. Thorofare, NJ: Slack.

Levitas, R. (1996). The concept of social exclusion and the new Durkheimian hegemony. *Critical Social Policy*, **16**, 5–20. doi: 10.1177/026101839601604601

Levitas, R. (1998). *The Inclusive Society? Social Exclusion and New Labour*. London: Macmillan Press.

Levitas, R., Pantazis, C., Fahmy, E. *et al.* (2007). *The multi-dimensional analysis of social exclusion*. Retrieved March 29, 2011, from http://citeseerx.ist.psu.edu/viewdoc/download?doi=10.1.1.127.339&rep=rep1&type=pdf

Lister, R. (1998). From equality to social inclusion: New Labour and the welfare state. *Critical Social Policy*, **18**, 215–25. doi: 10.1177/026101839801805505

Lister, R. (1999, June 9). Social exclusion: First steps to a fairer society. *The Guardian*, Society Pages, p. 2.

Lister, R. (2004). Defining poverty. In R. Lister (Ed.), *Poverty* (pp. 12–36). Cambridge: Polity Press.

Lister, R. (2010). *Just citizenship: Reflections on citizenship and social justice*. The Australian Social Policy Association (ASPA) Occasional Lecture series. Lecture. Australian Social Policy Association; Social Policy Research Centre; Social Policy Research Network. Sydney, New South Wales.

Lombe, M., & Sherraden, M. (2008). Inclusion in the policy process: An agenda for participation of the marginalized. *Journal of Policy Practice*, 7, 199–213. doi: 10.1080/15588740801938043

Luttrell, C., Quiroz, S., Scrutton, C., & Bird, K. (2009). *Understanding and Operationalising Empowerment*. Retrieved 4 April 2011, from http://www.odi.org.uk/resources/download/4525.pdf

Maulana, A. E., & Eckhardt, G. M. (2007). Just friends, good acquaintances or soul mates? An exploration of web site connectedness. *Qualitative Market Research: An International Journal*, **10**, 227–42.

Miller, D. (2011). *Saudi Women Suffer Setbacks as Conservatives Rise*. Retrieved 5 April 2011 from http://www.jpost.com/MiddleEast/Article.aspx?id=215138

Miller Polgar, J., & Landry, J.E. (2004). Occupations as a means for individual and group participation in life. In C.H. Christiansen & E.A. Townsend (Eds), *Introduction to Occupation: The Art and Science of Living* (pp. 197–220). Upper Saddle River, NJ: Pearson Education.

Mitchell, A., & Shillington, R. (2005). Poverty, inequality and social inclusion. In T. Richmond & A. Saloojee (Eds), *Social Inclusion: Canadian Perspectives* (pp. 33–57). Toronto: Laidlaw Foundation.

Molineux, M., & Whiteford, G. (2006). Occupational science: Genesis, evolution and future contribution. In E. Duncan (Ed.), *Foundations of Practice in Occupational Therapy* (pp. 295–312). London: Elsevier.

Morrison, Z. (2010). *On Dignity: Social Inclusion and the Politics of Recognition*. Melbourne, Victoria: Brotherhood of St Laurence.

Nelms, L., & Tsingas, C. (2010). *Literature Review on Social Inclusion and its Relationship to Minimum Wages and Workforce Participation*. Barton, Australian Capital Territory: Fair Work Victoria.

Nevile, A. (2007). Amartya K. Sen and social exclusion. *Development in Practice*, **17**, 249–55. doi: 10.1080/09614520701197200

Nussbaum, M. (2003). Capabilities as fundamental entitlements: Sen and social justice. *Feminist Economics*, **9**, 33–59. doi: 10.1080/1354570022000077926

Owens, J. (2009). The influence of 'access' on social exclusion and social connectedness for people with disabilities. In A. Taket, B. Crisp, G. Lamaro, M. Graham & S. Barter-Godfrey (Eds), *Theorising Social Exclusion* (pp. 78–86). Abingdon: Routledge.

Pettit, P. (2001). Symposium on Amartya Sen's philosophy: 1 Capability and freedom: A defence of Sen. *Economics and Philosophy*, **17**, 1–20.

Pieris, Y., & Craik, C. (2004). Factors enabling and hindering participation in leisure for people with mental health problems. *British Journal of Occupational Therapy*, **67**, 240–7.

Polatajko, H.J., Davis, J., Stewart, D. *et al.* (2007). Specifying the domain of concern: Occupation as core. In E.A. Townsend & Polatajko, H.J. (Eds). *Enabling Occupation II: Advancing an Occupational Therapy Vision for Health, Well-being, & Justice through Occupation* (pp. 13–36). Ottawa: CAOT Publications ACE.

Rawls, J. (1971). *A Theory of Justice*. Cambridge, MA: Harvard University Press.

Rawls, J. (1999). Justice as fairness: Political not metaphysical. In S. Freeman (Ed.), *John Rawls: Collected Papers*. Cambridge, MA: Harvard University Press.

Rebeiro, K.L. (2001). Enabling occupation: The importance of an affirming environment. *Canadian Journal of Occupational Therapy*, **68**, 80–9.

Reiter, S. (2008). *Disability from a Humanistic Perspective: Towards a Better Quality of Life*. New York, NY: Nova Science Publishers.

Renner, S., Prewitt, G., Watanabe, M., & Gascho, L. (2007). *Summary of the Virtual Round Table on Social Exclusion*. Retrieved 4 April 2011, from http://hdr.undp.org/en/nhdr/networks/replies/161.pdf

Saloojee, A. (2001). *Social Inclusion, Citizenship and Diversity*. Paper presented at the 'A new way of thinking? Towards a vision of social inclusion' conference, Ottawa, Canada. http://www.ccsd.ca/subsites/inclusion/bp/as.htm

Saloojee, A. (2005). Social inclusion, anti racism and democratic citizenship. In T. Richmond & A. Saloojee (Eds), *Social Inclusion: Canadian Perspectives* (pp. 180–202). Toronto: Laidlaw Foundation.

Saloojee, A. (2011). *Social Inclusion: Theory and Practice over 2 Continents*. Paper presented at the Inclusive Futures Conference, Sydney, Australia.

Saunders, P. (2003). *Can Social Exclusion Provide a New Framework for Measuring Poverty?* Sydney, NSW: Social Policy Research Centre.

Saunders, P., Naidoo, Y., & Griffiths, M. (2007). *Towards New Indicators of disadvantage: Deprivation and Social Exclusion in Australia*. Sydney, NSW: Social Policy Research Centre.

Sayce, L. (2001). Social inclusion and mental health. [Editorial]. *Psychiatric Bulletin*, **25**, 121–3.

Sen, A. (1992). *Inequality Reexamined*. Oxford: Oxford University Press.

Sen, A. (1993). Capability and well-being. In A. Sen & M. Nussbaum (Eds), *The Quality of Life* (pp. 30–53). Oxford: Oxford University Press.

Sen, A. (1999). *Development as Freedom*. Oxford: Oxford University Press.

Sen, A. (2000). *Social Exclusion: Concept, Application, and Scrutiny. Social Development Papers No. 1*. Manila, Philippines: Asian Development Bank.

Sen, A. (2001). Symposium on Amartya Sen's philosophy: 4 – Reply. *Economics and Philosophy*, **17**, 51–66.

Sen, A. (2004). Capabilities, lists, and public reason: Continuing the conversation. *Feminist Economics*, **10**, 77–80. doi: 10.1080/1354570042000315163

Sen, A., & Nussbaum, M. (Eds). (1993). *The Quality of Life*. Oxford: Oxford University Press.

Shakespeare, T. (2006). *Disability Rights and Wrongs*. Abingdon: Routledge.

Shergold, P. (2009). Social inclusion: An agenda for citizen empowerment. *Australian Philanthropy*, **74**, 5–7.

Sinclair, S., Bramley, G., Dobbie, L., & Gillespie, M. (2007). *Social inclusion and communications: A review of the literature*. Retrieved 11 March 2011, from http://www.communicationsconsumerpanel.org.uk/downloads/Research/LowIncomeConsumers_Research/Social%20inclusion%20and%20communications/Social%20inclusion%20and%20communications.pdf

Silver, H. (1994). Social exclusion and social solidarity: Three paradigms. *International Labour Review*, **133**, 531–78.

Smith, S. R. (2009). Social justice and disability: Competing interpretations of the medical and social model. In K. Kristiansen, S. Vehmas & T. Shakespeare (Eds), *Arguing about Disability: Philosophical Perspectives* (pp. 15–29). Abingdon: Routledge.

Smyth, P. (2008). *Social Inclusion and Place Based Disadvantage: The Australian Context*. Melbourne: Brotherhood of St Laurence.

Smyth, P. (2010). *In or Out? Building an Inclusive Nation*. Melbourne: Brotherhood of St Laurence.

Social Exclusion Task Force. (2009). *What do We Mean by Social Exclusion?* Retrieved 27 March 2010, from http://www.cabinetoffice.gov.uk/social_exclusion_task_force/context/

Stadnyk, R.L., Townsend, E.A., & Wilcock, A.A. (2010). Occupational justice. In C.H. Christiansen & E.A. Townsend (Eds), *Introduction to Occupation: The Art and Science of Living* (2nd ed., pp. 328–58). Upper Saddle River, NJ: Pearson Education.

Stephens, U. (2010). *A Fair Go or Fair Enough – What does a Socially Inclusive Australia Look Like?* Paper presented at the Social Inclusion Conference, Melbourne, Victoria, Australia.

Strong, S., Rigby, P., Stewart, D. *et al.* (1999). Application of the Person-Environment-Occupation Model: A practical tool. *Canadian Journal of Occupational Therapy*, **66**, 122–33.

Taket, A., Crisp, B.R., Nevill, A. *et al.* (Eds). (2009). *Theorising Social Exclusion*. Abingdon: Routledge.

Terzi, L. (2009). Vagaries of the natural lottery? Human diversity, disability, and justice: A capability perspective. In K. Brownlee & A. Cureton (Eds), *Disability and Disadvantage* (pp. 86–111). Oxford: Oxford University Press.

Townsend, E., & Brintnell, S. (1997). Context of occupational therapy. In E. Townsend (Ed.), *Enabling Occupation: An Occupational Therapy Perspective* (pp. 9–28). Ottawa: CAOT Publications ACE.

Townsend, K.C., & McWhirter, B.T. (2005). Connectedness: A review of the literature with implications for counseling, assessment, and research. *Journal of Counseling & Development*, **83**, 191–201.

Tutu, D. (1999). *No Future without Forgiveness*. New York, NY: Random House.
United Nations (UN). (1948). *Universal Declaration of Human Rights*. Retrieved 5 April 2011, from http://www.udhr.org/udhr/udhr.HTM
Vasta, E. (2010a). The controllability of difference: Social cohesion and the new politics of solidarity. *Ethnicities*, **10**, 503–21. doi: 10.1177/1468796810378326
Vasta, E. (2010b). *Solidarity and Social Inclusion*. Paper presented at the Concepts of Social Inclusion Workshop Series, Centre for Research on Social Inclusion, Macquarie University, Sydney, Australia.
Vasta, E. (2011). *Migration and Solidarity: The Changing Fashions of Inclusionary Concepts*. Paper presented at the Inclusive Futures Conference, Sydney, Australia.
Vinson, T. (2007). *Dropping Off the Edge: The Distribution of Disadvantage in Australia*. Richmond, Vic.: Jesuit Social Services/Catholic Social Services Australia.
Vinson, T. (2009). *Markedly Social Disadvantaged Localities in Australia: Their Nature and Possible Remediation*. Barton, Australian Capital Territory: Commonwealth of Australia.
Ward, N. (2009). Social exclusion, social identity and social work: Analysing social exclusion from a material discursive perspective. *Social Work Education*, **28**, 237–52. doi: 10.1080/02615470802659332
Whiteford, G. (2000). Occupational deprivation: Global challenge in the new millennium. *British Journal of Occupational Therapy*, **63**, 200–4.
Whiteford, G., & Townsend, E. (2011). Participatory occupational justice framework (POJF 2010): Enabling occupational participation and inclusion. In F. Kronenberg, N. Pollard & D. Sakellariou (Eds), *Occupational Therapies without Borders: Towards an Ecology of Occupation-based Practices* (Vol. 2, pp. 65–84). London: Elsevier.
Whiteford, G., & Wright-St Clair, V. (Eds). (2005). *Occupation and Practice in Context*. Marrickville, NSW: Elsevier Australia.
Wilcock, A.A. (2006). *An Occupational Perspective of Health* (2nd ed.). Thorofare, NJ: Slack.
World Health Organization (WHO). (1998). *Health Promotion Glossary*. Retrieved 4 April 2011, from http://www.who.int/hpr/NPH/docs/hp_glossary_en.pdf
World Health Organization (WHO). (2008). *Closing the Gap in a Generation: Health Equity through Action on the Social Determinants of Health. Final Report of the Commission on Social Determinants of Health*. Geneva: World Health Organization.

Index

Occupational Science: Society, Inclusion, Participation, First Edition.
Edited by Gail Whiteford and Clare Hocking.

Printed and bound by CPI Group (UK) Ltd, Croydon, CR0 4YY

27/10/2024

14580396-0001